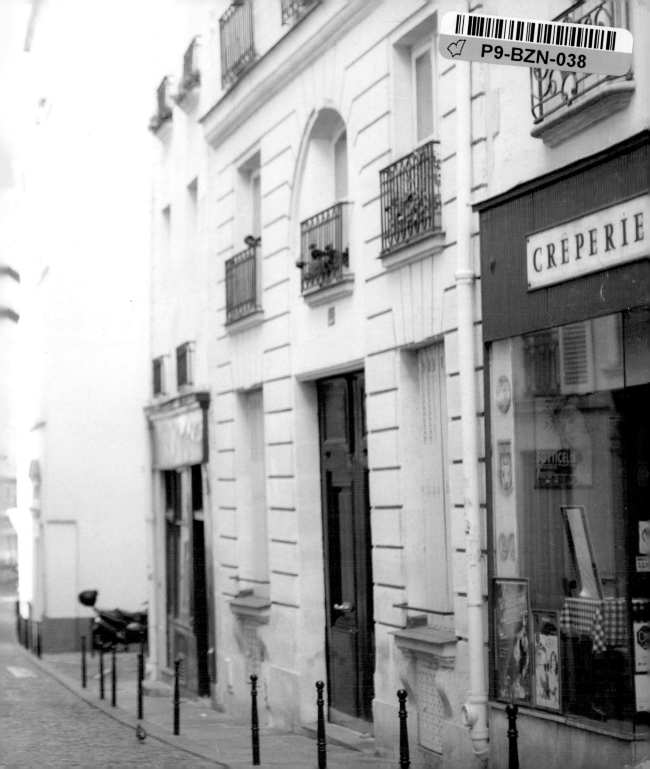

CRÊPERIE

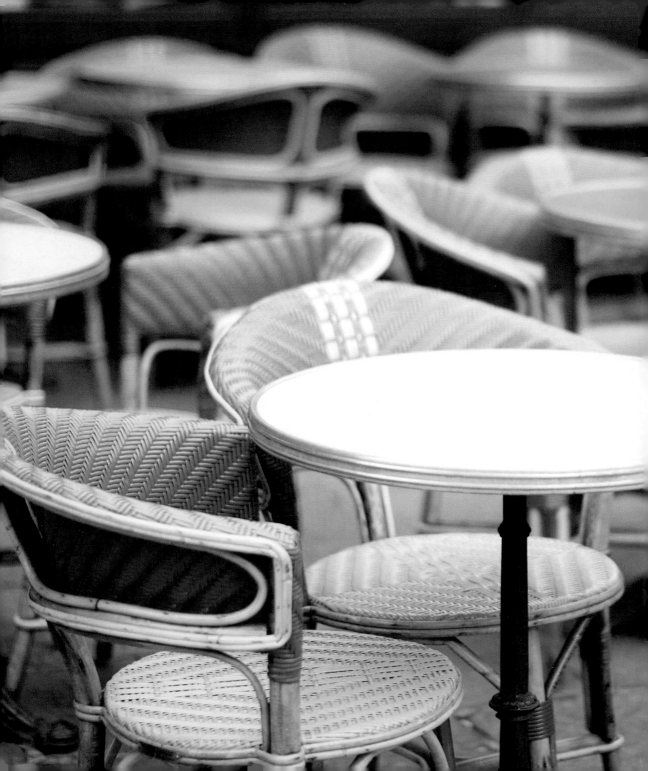

Bright Lights Paris

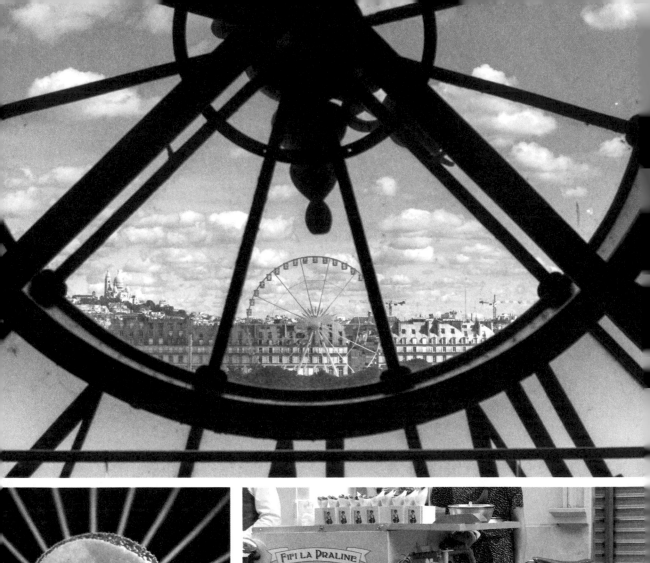

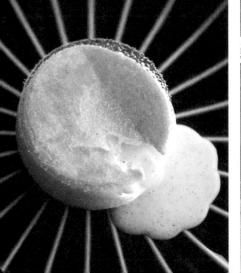

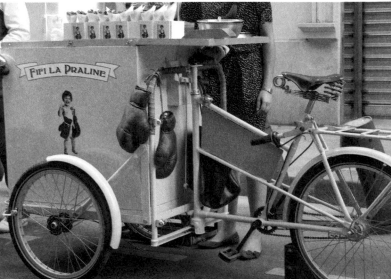

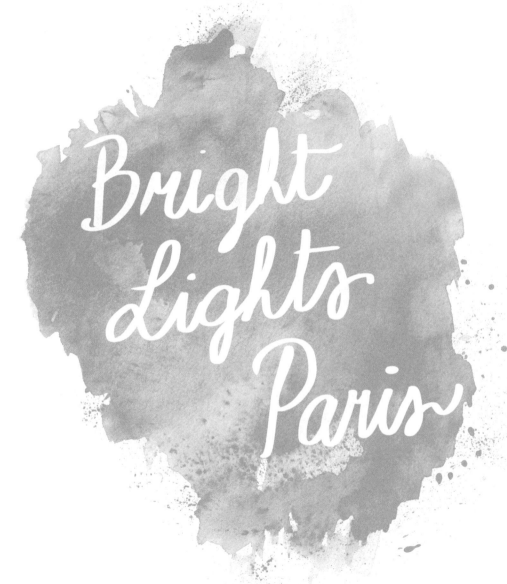

Bright Lights Paris

ANGIE NILES

BERKLEY BOOKS, NEW YORK

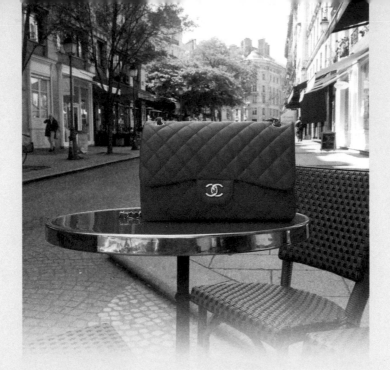

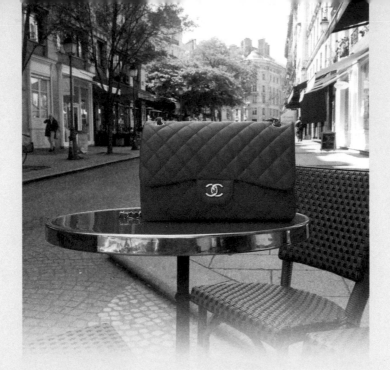

Berkley
An imprint of Penguin Random House LLC
375 Hudson Street, New York, New York 10014

Copyright © 2015 by Angie Niles.

A list of photo credits appears on page 289.

For more information, visit penguin.com.

ISBN: 978-0-425-28070-6

An application for cataloging has been submitted to the Library of Congress.

PUBLISHING HISTORY
Berkley trade paperback edition / September 2015

PRINTED IN THE UNITED STATES OF AMERICA

10 9 8 7 6 5 4 3 2 1

Cover photos: (front) © Jason McDonald
(back) Haleigh Walsworth.
Interior text design by Georgia Rucker.

Penguin
Random
House

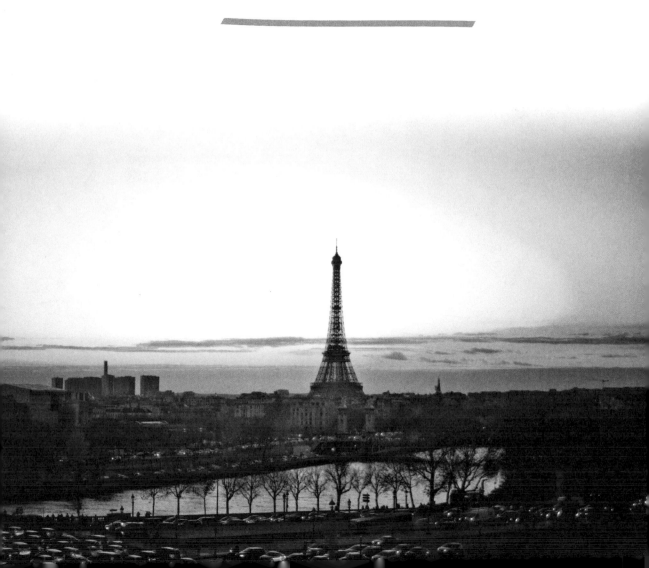

To *Penny*

Your chic Parisian spirit is like no one else! Stay cute and stay French!

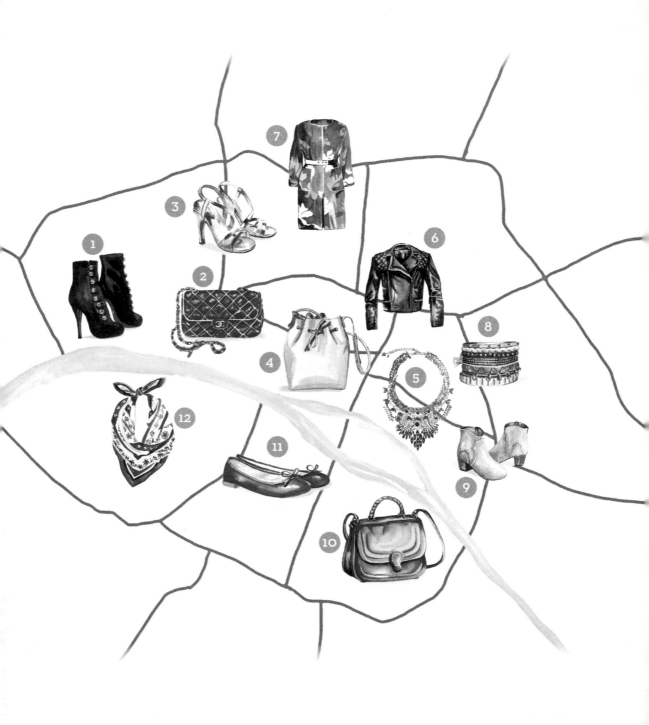

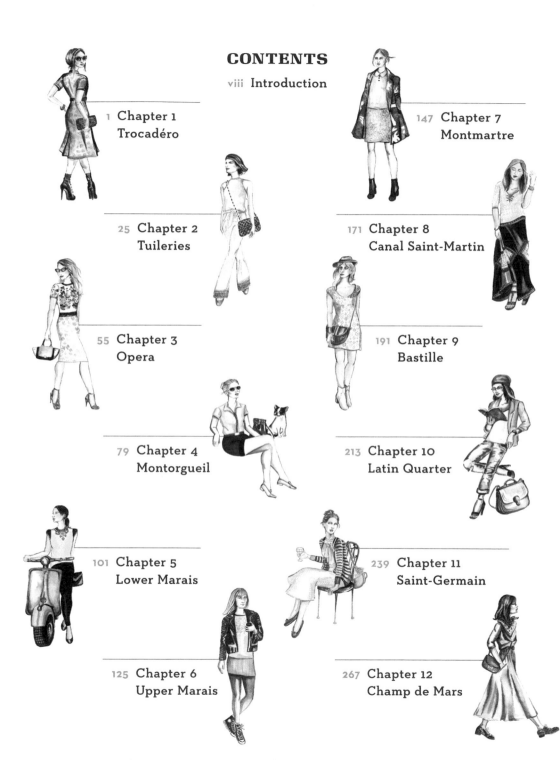

CONTENTS

viii Introduction

1 Chapter 1
Trocadéro

25 Chapter 2
Tuileries

55 Chapter 3
Opera

79 Chapter 4
Montorgueil

101 Chapter 5
Lower Marais

125 Chapter 6
Upper Marais

147 Chapter 7
Montmartre

171 Chapter 8
Canal Saint-Martin

191 Chapter 9
Bastille

213 Chapter 10
Latin Quarter

239 Chapter 11
Saint-Germain

267 Chapter 12
Champ de Mars

INTRODUCTION

Paris Is Beautiful.
Paris Is Charming.
Paris Is Enchanting.
Paris Is . . . Magical.

When I lived in Paris, I would wake each morning to the bells of Notre Dame reminding me that I wasn't just dreaming about Paris but actually living there. Walking along the cobblestone streets, I discovered so many magical places and experienced all that this special city has to offer: open-air food markets with seasonal fresh vegetables and mounds of Camembert cheese ready to drip out onto your warm, crusty baguette; sensational restaurants delighting taste buds you didn't even know you had; unique boutiques carrying the most intricately detailed baubles; manicured parks perfect for picnicking; and most important, the city's residents, with a Parisian style and character all their own.

My first introduction to the City of Lights, however, was not on rue de Rivoli. Like many others, it started from afar, by first seeing the city's beauty in movies like *Breathless*, *A Little Romance*, and *Charade*, with the ever-so-chic Audrey Hepburn. I was also

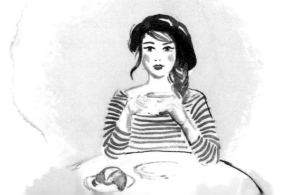

lucky to have grown up near Disney World in Central Florida, with a petite Paris at Epcot. My mom and I had yearly passes from the time I was a kid until I finished college. Whenever we were shopping in Orlando, she would say, "Let's go have dessert in Paris," and we would drive to Epcot, stop by "Paris" for chocolate croissants or a gooey Napoleon pastry, and sit outside at their replica Parisian café.

This was the closest my mom or I had ever been to Paris. I loved the "mini" version so much, that I often found myself daydreaming of traveling to the real City of Lights and wondering what a Parisian girl's life was like—how she lived, what she wore, who she was.

It wasn't until college that I took my first trip to Paris. And it was while walking around Le Marais that I first encountered her: the Parisian Girl. There were women heading to the market for their weekly groceries, ladies looking impossibly chic as they browsed the modern art galleries and designer boutiques, and young women gathered at outdoor cafés sipping their café au lait with friends.

With every trip my fascination grew, and it soon became clear there was not just one type of woman in Paris, but more than a dozen . . . that Parisian girls from each arrondissement have their own unique sense of style and way of life. I was intrigued and delighted by their lively differences. From girls in Canal Saint-Martin wandering along the canal with a bohemian spirit, to the perfectly put together ladies in Saint-Germain-des-Prés who shop the art galleries and meet up for lunch at Café de Flore. And let's not forget the eclectic artists in Montmartre and the chic modern styles of the ladies who ride their Vespas through the streets of the Marais.

Now, after living in Paris and many trips there since, I'm here to share everything I have learned with you. Join me through the life of Parisian women. We'll go shopping with them to eclectic vintage shops, take weekend excursions to nearby vineyards, share their beauty secrets, and learn about the hidden gems only a true Parisian knows how to find. Whether you are planning a trip to Paris, dreaming of one from your living room, or just aspiring to live like a Parisian, *Bright Lights Paris* will show you the way.

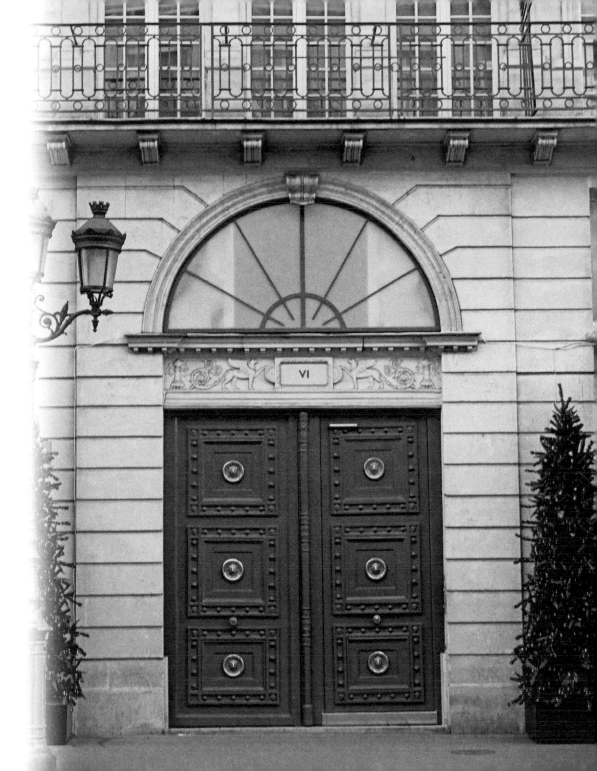

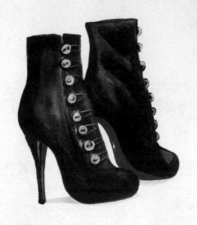

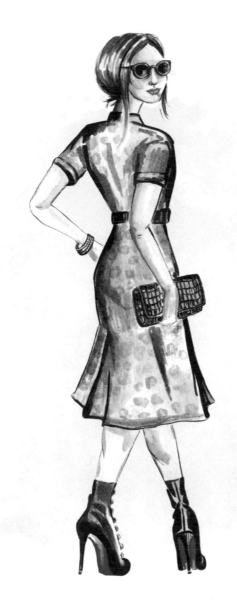

CHAPTER 1
TROCADÉRO

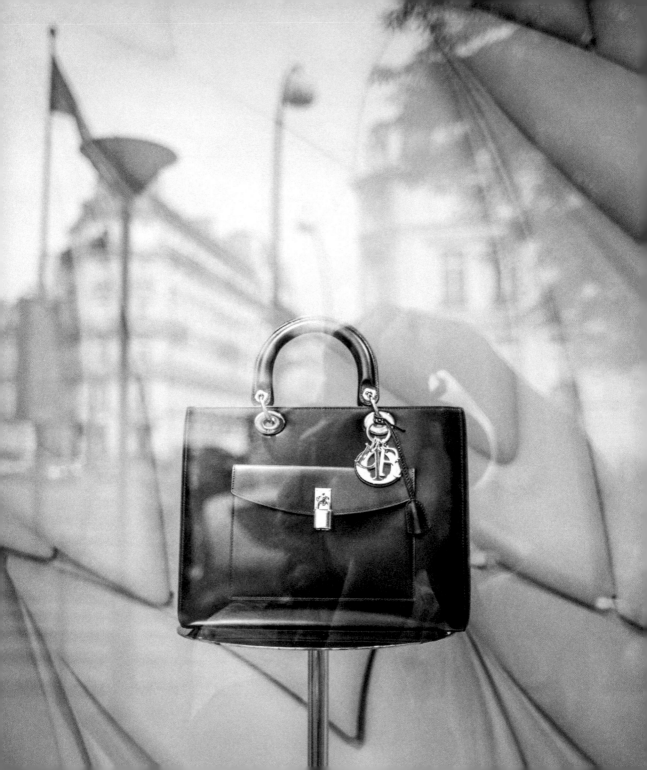

In the world that is Trocadéro in Paris's 16th arrondissement, wide tree-lined boulevards lead the way for the well-heeled elite to haute couture and haute cuisine. The epitome of French bourgeoisie chic, the Trocadéro woman attends designer boutique openings, strolls past elegant couture houses on her way to work, and sips tea at the Hôtel Plaza Athénée, where Carrie Bradshaw stayed with Aleksandr Petrovsky.

With a closet full of high-end luxury labels, her daytime elegance shines in Lanvin and Erdem dresses paired with a Vanessa Bruno tuxedo blazer. When she's in the mood for rock 'n' roll chic, the Trocadéro woman slips into her Balmain army jacket and tapered pants, or fitted bias-cut miniskirt by Jay Ahr. For black-tie affairs, only a Saint Laurent draped gown will do.

Red-soled Christian Louboutin stilettos are her wardrobe staple and line the closet of her pied-à-terre, which is attached to her family's nineteenth-century mansion. For handbags, she has curated a collection of standout luxury pieces in classic colors—red, black, navy, and brown—by Givenchy, Céline, and Saint Laurent. When her mom needs new pieces for her wardrobe, they shop at Guy Laroche and Nina Ricci, followed by lunch at the Four Seasons Hotel George V.

Not only does she possess a luxury wardrobe, but she also lives the life of luxury. On weekends, she can be found brunching at Carette on the Place du Trocadéro, then strolling through the elegant Park Monceau surrounded by luxury town houses and former homes of writers Colette and Proust on rue de Courcelles. Raised on bubbly, she frequents the Avenue de Champagne for tastings at the world's most famous champagne houses in the nearby town of Épernay.

She shares her neighborhood with the most famous couple in Paris, Fa-raon and Kléopatre, the Burmese felines who live and welcome guests at Hôtel Le Bristol. One thing she won't admit is that on occasion, she and her boyfriend head to her secret spot and sit on a wall with a bottle of champagne to watch the Eiffel Tower sparkle. With no cars passing by or tourists taking photos, the two enjoy a quiet Parisian evening alone.

She steps foot on the Champs-Élysées for three reasons and three reasons only: to shop last-minute pharmacy necessities on Sunday since nothing else nearby is open, to meet friends at the movies, and for her favorite facials at Biologique Recherche.

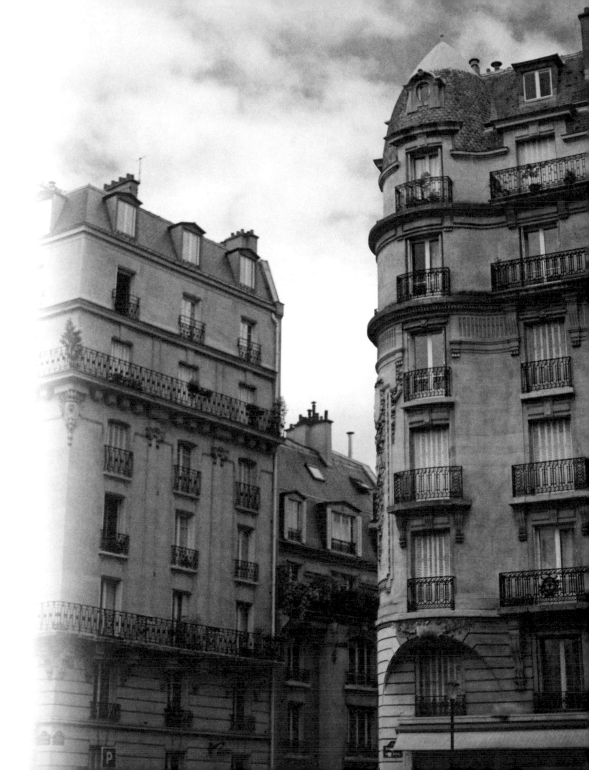

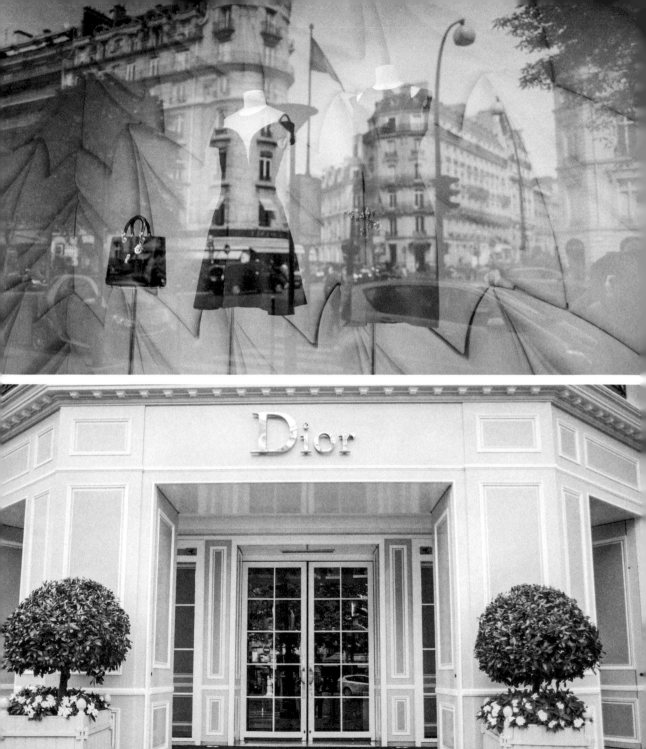

LE TRIANGLE D'OR

A small part of this arrondissement has been dubbed "The Golden Triangle." Here you'll find the finest couture houses and cafés surrounded by the perfect triangle formed by Avenue Montaigne, Avenue George V, and Avenue des Champs-Élysées.

Artcurial
7, Rond Point Des Champs-Élysées

A beautiful town house with the largest collection of art books in Paris. Along with eighteen thousand titles you'll find art exhibitions, a café, and an art auction house. Check the auction schedule and watch firsthand how Trocadéro women buy their art and vintage estate jewelry.

Montaigne Market
57, Avenue Montaigne

This designer concept boutique curates a selection of cutting-edge contemporary collections for men and women. Known for helping launch some of the most talented up-and-coming designers in Europe, it's a Trocadéro girl's first stop for new designer jeans, perfect-fitting T-shirts, or an exceptionally chic dress.

Céline
53, Avenue Montaigne

This French ready-to-wear brand has re-emerged as a force in the luxury handbag market with their more recent styles, the Luggage Tote and Trapeze bag.

L'avenue
41, Avenue Montaigne

Inside it's a chic scene of fashion power lunches, and out on the terrace you'll find relaxed Parisians enjoying their meal in the sunshine. Be on the lookout for A-listers like Jay-Z and Beyoncé. Not just a who's-who lunch spot; the food is also delicious.

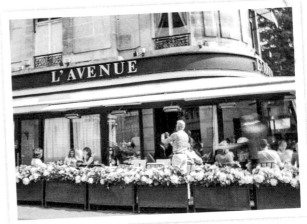

Christian Dior
30, Avenue Montaigne

The House of Dior's couture atelier and first boutique is full of fashion history. It set the scene for the debut of Dior's "New Look" in 1947, a dreamy Jean Seberg gazing into the boutique in Godard's *Breathless*, and the epic fall Carrie Bradshaw took in the final episode of *Sex and the City*.

Hôtel Plaza Athénée
25, Avenue Montaigne

The luxury palace hotel welcomes you with their trademark red awnings and flowers at every window—and a breathtaking view of the Eiffel Tower. During an afternoon of shopping, Trocadéro girls stop by the terrace café for tea or a glass of wine. When they have a special occasion to celebrate, Chef Alain Ducasse's eponymous three-Michelin-star gastronomy delights them with a dazzling meal.

Louis Vuitton
22, Avenue Montaigne

Parisians skip the tourist-filled flagship on the Champs-Élysées and instead shop at Louis Vuitton's much quieter gem on Montaigne for their ready-to-wear, signature handbags, and leather goods.

Le Stresa
7, Rue Chambiges

Owned and run by a family of six Italian brothers, this trattoria serves delicious pastas and seafood to the chicest Parisian socialites and filmmakers.

Givenchy
3, Avenue George V

Creative director Riccardo Tisci has revived this couture house with his infusion of gothic touches and chic modernism. Trocadéro women love every piece from his ready-to-wear collection and signature accessories.

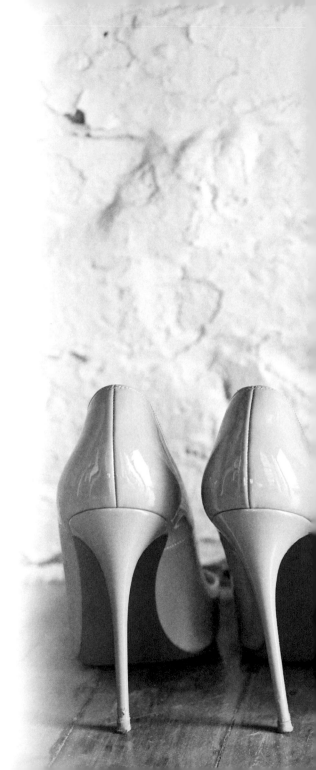

—Jamie Chung, **ACTRESS AND FOUNDER OF WHATTHECHUNG.COM**

I can't help but fall more in love with Paris every time I visit. Similar to when I am in New York City, I just put in my earphones and walk. I walk along the water, over the Bridge of Locked Hearts, through the Jardin des Plantes and under the Eiffel Tower. I'll usually find a café selected at random and stop for a latte and people watch. I can do this for hours! What I can't leave Paris without doing is shopping near the Champs-Élysées—which means sometimes splurging on one chic French accessory!

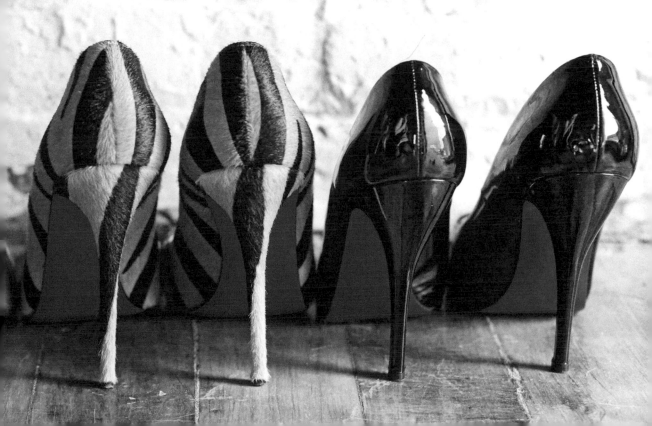

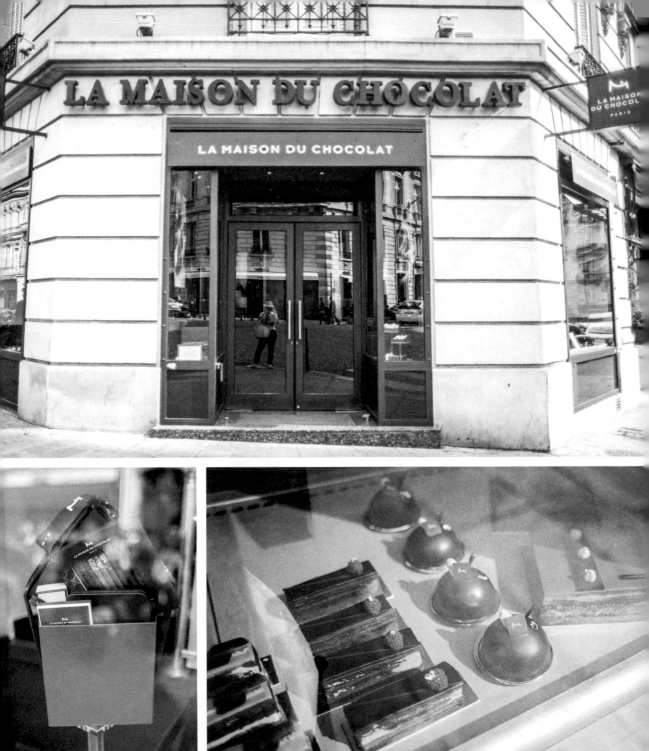

Balenciaga
10, Avenue George V

Trocadéro girls' go-to for rock 'n' roll glamour. You'll find motorcycle-inspired details on everything from handbags and boots to leather jackets and cashmere sweaters.

Maison de la Truffe
14, Rue Marbeuf

When it comes to food, there aren't many ingredients more decadent than fresh white or black truffles shaved onto a dish of creamy linguini pasta or seared halibut. Trocadéro ladies stop in for lunch or to pick up gourmet truffle gifts for a friend's housewarming party.

La Maison du Chocolate
52, Rue François 1er

Chocolate cravings take her to no other location than La Maison du Chocolate. Although there is an array of decadent choices, it's their creamy and luxurious dark chocolate truffles dusted in cocoa powder that keep her coming back time and again.

Balmain
44, Rue François 1er

French women have never looked so chic than when wearing both army jackets and couture gowns by the House of Balmain. Creative director Olivier Rousteing has proven that, even at a young age, he's a force to be reckoned with.

Courrèges
40, Rue François 1er

This futuristically designed space, opened in 1965, continues to sell their collection of signature go-go miniskirts and shift dresses.

La Maison de L'aubrac
37, Rue Marbeuf

Stop by for a late dinner at this nightly gathering place for chefs and night owls. Known for signature steak dishes, the owner receives high-quality beef from his family cattle farm in the countryside region of Aubrac.

Wolford
39, Rue Marbeuf

Trocadéro women shop here for sexy tights, shapewear, and bodysuits. Parisian women like to accentuate their best features, not hide them.

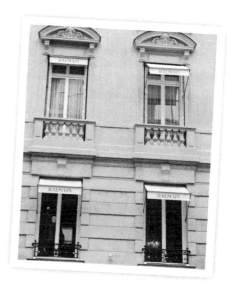

A WORTHY SPLURGE

The first luxury bag in my petite collection of designer pieces was from the one and only Chanel. A joint birthday gift from a few friends, receiving it was a pivotal moment in the life of my wardrobe. I know it's just an "item," but it's still a special piece I will always love. It takes a team of skilled ladies to make these beautiful bags, down to their hand weaving of the leather-and-metal-woven straps. Their attention to detail is flawless. I joke that a girl's first Chanel is sometimes more memorable than her first love. For my navy-blue satchel and me, that's definitely the case.

French women do not buy luxury handbags on a regular basis. They splurge and build a small collection of handbags in timeless shapes and colors that can be carried throughout the year.

The Trocadéro woman might buy the current popular shape or silhouette, just not in the cobalt blue or burgundy/gold python. Instead she'll select classic colors like solid natural brown, black, navy, or red. Parisians are skilled in predicting which "it bag" silhouettes will become the new timeless classics—like Givenchy's Antigona satchel, Céline's Trapeze tote, and the Saint Laurent Sac de Jour tote. While these bags are very "of the moment," it's only a matter of a few years before each will be considered a classic wardrobe piece.

My friend Helena bases her designer splurges on "cost per wear," often mentioning the term on her chic lifestyle blog, *Brooklyn Blonde*. She doesn't mind spending extra on classic pieces she will wear so much more often than less expensive pieces, which tend to wear out or go out of style. It's a great tip to think about when considering a splurge for your wardrobe.

While a luxury bag is not always an everyday accessory, that doesn't mean you can take it out only a few times a year for special occasions. What would be the point in that? You'll enjoy her even more when she joins you on date night or dinner with your girlfriends. Take good care of her, but remember she's not there to be left on a shelf.

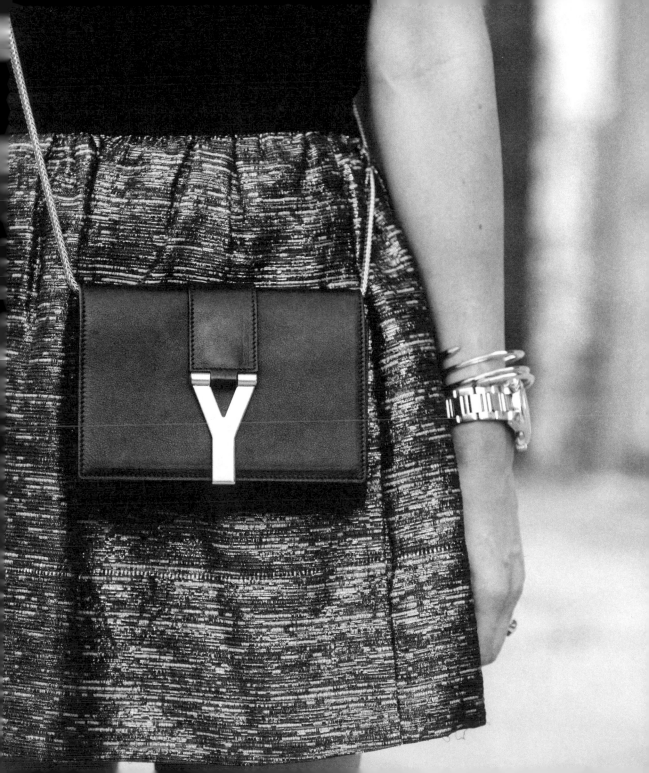

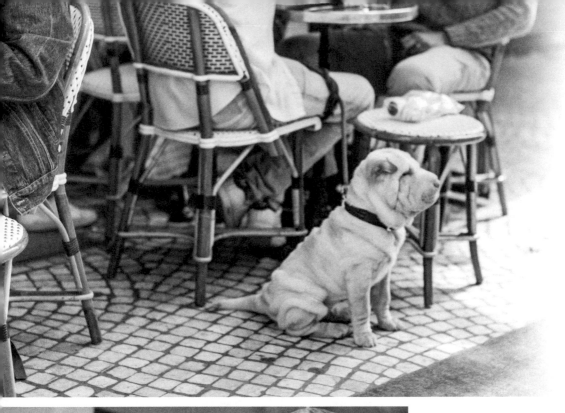

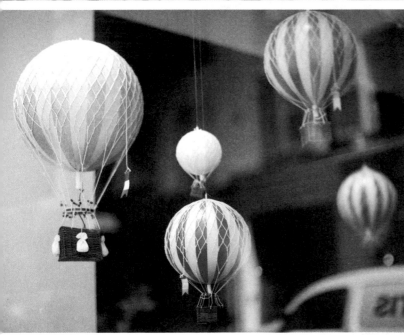

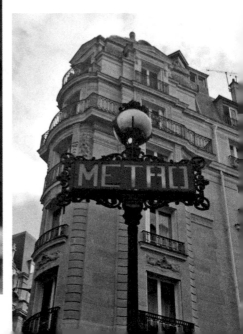

Fondation Pierre Bergé, Yves St Laurent
5, Avenue Marceau

YSL's former couture house and atelier were converted into a museum, research library, and exhibition space set up by his partner Pierre Bergé. The collection archives include five thousand couture pieces and more than fifteen thousand accessories. It's a dreamy and elegant journey through Saint Laurent's life and collections.

Palais Galliera Fashion Museum
10, Avenue Pierre 1er de Serbie

This museum hosts temporary fashion exhibits on costume and clothing design from the eighteenth century to present. For Paris fashionistas, the nineteenth-century garden is the place to be seen on opening day of the exhibits.

Palais de Tokyo
13, Avenue du Président Wilson

Parisians love the mix of art, music, and science in the avant-garde modern art exhibitions that are held in this art nouveau palace. Dine at the museum's newest restaurant, Monsieur Bleu, for lunch or late- night drinks with friends, looking out at a scenic view of the river Seine. It's exceptionally spectacular to see at sunset.

Maison Baccarat
11, Place des Etats-Unis

This Philippe Starck–designed flagship with oversized crystal furniture and chess sets would be the perfect French playground for Alice in Wonderland. It's a great place for a special girls' lunch, but don't forget to dress to impress.

Saint James Paris
43, Avenue Bugeaud

When they need an escape without leaving the city, the Trocadéro ladies head to the only château hotel in Paris. Whether they are enjoying brunch and a glass of rosé champagne in the dreamy garden, tea in the library bar, or a full day of pampering at Le Spa Guerlain, they can always be sure of a decadent day.

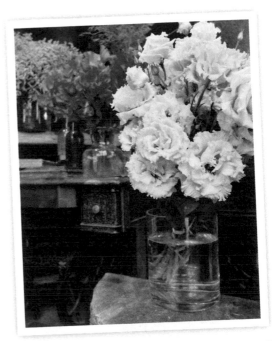

A BUBBLY DAY TRIP

What's better than a bottle of champagne on Avenue Montaigne? An afternoon of tastings in the French Champagne region, of course. A Trocadéro girl loves a life of luxury, and there's nothing quite as luxurious as a glass of bubbly champagne. Especially when she's sipping on her glass in a mansion on the avenue de Champagne in Épernay. When she wants an escape from Paris, Épernay is her first choice for an afternoon of bubbly and fine dining. She travels the hour and a half by train or sometimes with a private car and driver—never having a friend drive, to prevent anyone in her group from being bored as the designated driver.

The Trocadéro woman most often visits the famous "couture" houses of champagne—Moët & Chandon, Perrier-Jouët, and Mercier—who host tours and tastings in their private mansions on the avenue de Champagne. When she wants a more in-depth experience visiting the vineyards and farms where the grapes are grown on-site, she'll visit Abel Jobart and Alfred Tritant for their Grand Cru bubbly.

Moët & Chandon has just completed a yearlong renovation of their cellars, making the champagne house's informative tours and tastings even more memorable. Trocadéro ladies may enjoy the VIP lounge with a personal butler serving them bubbly.

One of the most special and unique experiences a Trocadéro woman may have access to is a tour of Perrier-Jouët's Maison Belle Epoque. The former home of the Perrier family is now home to an incredible art museum and a residence for VIP clients to stay a night or two. It contains a private collection of two hundred art nouveau pieces that is the largest in Europe. When you arrive for your tour, ask if you too can visit the museum. If it's not currently in use, they may let you take a peek.

If you'd like to follow along in the footsteps of the Louboutin-heeled Trocadéro ladies but want to skip planning the day yourself, let the wine experts at O Chateau lead the way. With a small guided tour, you will enjoy a scenic ride through the beautiful countryside east of Paris, visit both large houses in Épernay and some of the smaller, family-run vineyards near Reims, such as Penet-Chardonnet and Nicolas Maillart. Learn how champagne is made, all the while tasting amazing champagne both at lunch and at the wineries.

Moët & Chandon, 20, Avenue de Champagne
Perrier-Jouët, 26, Avenue de Champagne
Mercier, 70, Avenue de Champagne
Nicolas Maillart, 5, Rue de Villers, Écueil
Penet-Chardonnet, 4, Rue Arthur Lallement, Verzy

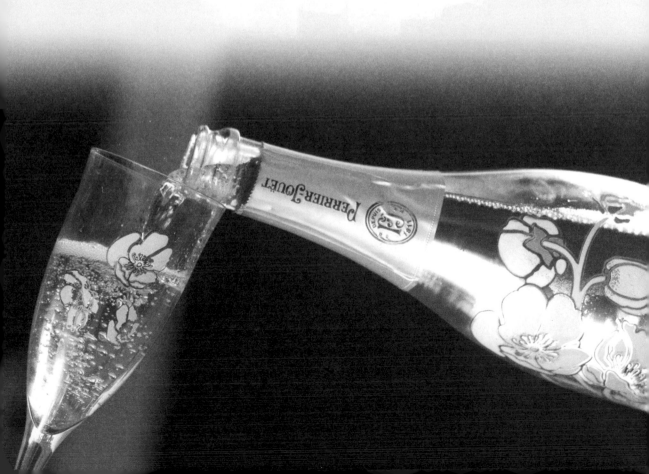

MICHELIN STARS

Trocadéro women are blessed not only with being surrounded by elegant couture houses but also with having more Michelin-starred restaurants in their arrondissement than the rest of Paris combined. Along with the palace hotel greats at Plaza Athénée, Le Bristol, and George V, here are just a few of the others near her with extraordinary dishes.

L'ASTRANCE, 4 Rue Beethoven

Fruit and vegetables reign supreme on Chef Pascale Barbot's seasonal tasting menus. His haute cuisine is inventive and whimsical, and the three Michelin stars are beyond well deserved.

RESTAURANT PIERRE GAGNAIRE, 6, Rue Balzac

Chef Pierre Gagnaire and his three Michelin stars take diners on a bold culinary journey of contrasting flavors, textures, and colors. His first course arrives as five to six mini plates at once, and his signature Grand Dessert is just . . . grand.

APICIUS, 20, Rue d'Artois

Two-Michelin-star chef Jean-Pierre Vigato showcases his cuisine in a lovely nineteenth-century Hotel Particulier. When the weather is warm you can dine in the garden and feel like you're miles away from the center of Paris.

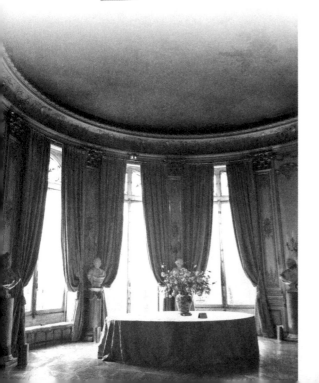

Musée Jacquemart-André
158, Boulevard Haussmann

Catch a glimpse of nineteenth-century bourgeoisie living in this extravagant mansion that Edouard André built in 1875 for himself and his wife Nélie Jacquemart. Now a museum, it showcases the paintings and other treasures they bought around the world together. I love their juxtaposed take on art, which mixes conservative religious-themed pieces with paintings and sculptures that have a naughty undertone.

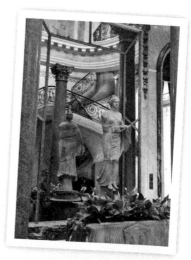

Caffè Burlot
9, Rue du Colisée

Feel the spirit of Italy in the 1950s at this Costes brothers' eatery. Fresh, simple Italian dishes done to perfection with a chic retro vibe. Let your imagination run away and you may just see Don Draper pass by.

Market
15, Avenue Matignon

Jean-George Vongerichten's first Paris restaurant with inventive fusion cuisine in an elegant (but not too fancy) setting. The simple, chic décor in neutral tones lets the eclectic Asian-French menu shine.

Grand and Petit Palais
Avenue Winston-Churchill and Cours la Reine

The beaux arts–style exhibition hall and museum are home to yearly art exhibitions and the best fashion shows each season. Chanel has transformed this space into amazing theatrical worlds, including a Chanel grocery store, a city setting with a women's-rights march, and even an "Under the Sea" world fit for mermaids. Both buildings are stunning, with glass vaulted ceilings and an iron frame. Trocadéro ladies in need of a late-night bite enjoy the terrace café at the Petit Palais.

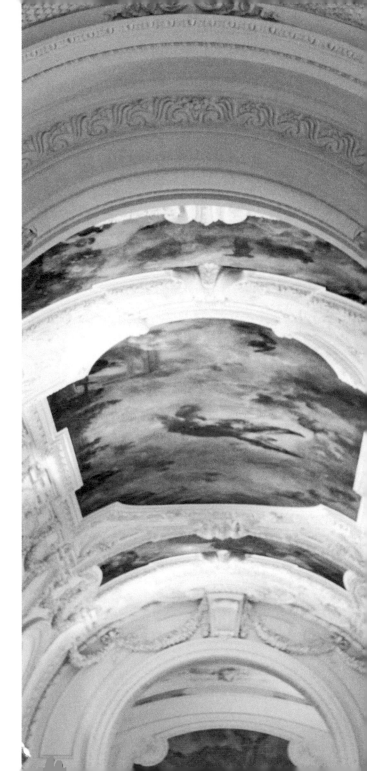

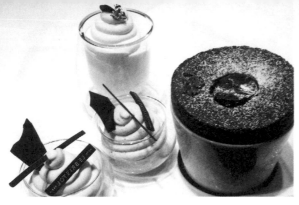

Les 110 de Taillevent
195, Rue du Faubourg Saint-Honoré

The brasserie of the Michelin-starred Taillevent specializes in wine pairings with 110 wines from their vault. They offer four wine pairings per dish in different size glasses and a range of prices. The Turbot Meunière in Beurre Blanc sauce is enough for two to three people to share. Just be warned, with a sauce so tasty you will definitely be fighting over the last bite.

Les Caves Taillevent
228, Rue du Faubourg Saint-Honoré

This wine shop sells only French-made wine and champagne. Trocadéro ladies stop by on Saturday afternoon for tastings of new selections and to stock their wine cellar at home.

Marché aux Timbres
Champs-Élysées (at the corner of avenues Gabriel and Marigny)

The old stamp market, where you can buy and trade vintage stamps, has been open a few days a week for more than fifty years. Take a walk through and feel like you're back in time and on set of *Charade* with Cary Grant and Audrey Hepburn.

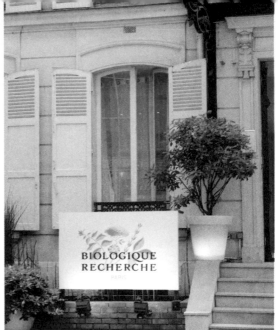

Hôtel Le Bristol
112, Rue du Faubourg Saint-Honoré

Le Bristol is a spectacular old world–style palace hotel. It's the first choice for a Trocadéro woman to bring visiting family for afternoon tea or to go for a quiet date night at the cocktail bar with her beau. Dine at Epicure, the formal three Michelin–starred gastronomique by Chef Eric Frechon, or downstairs at 114 Faubourg, the one-star luxury brasserie. Please don't leave without ordering the chocolate soufflé with cognac ice cream. It's absolutely the most amazing chocolate soufflé I have ever tasted. The hotel is also home to the most famous feline couple in Paris, Fa-aron and Kléopatre, who live and wander the hotel together. If you stop by, tell them I say hello.

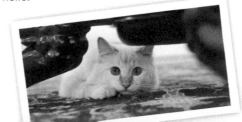

FIRST-CLASS SKIN CARE

Only once have I been lucky enough to experience an upgrade to first class on a flight to Paris. Not just any first-class experience, but on Air France no less. It was there, while wrapped in my cozy red blanket, that I was handed a chic toiletry kit and first used a Biologique face cream. As I've since learned from Parisian girlfriends, this isn't just any cream. It's the platinum Dom Pérignon of skin care.

Parisian woman focus more on skin care than makeup. For most, the makeup routine is simply a statement red lipstick and mascara. They may not spend as much time or money as American ladies do on certain beauty treatments, like manicures and pedicures, but they do spend money on their skin care routine and treatments. Sure, they also buy some of the less expensive French pharmacy brands, but they don't mind spending more on the products necessary to having and keeping incredibly healthy skin. To them, it's not just a luxury but a necessity to keep their skin looking and feeling fresh year-round.

They know the key to better-looking skin is having healthy skin. So it's not surprising that the only reason some Trocadéro women would dare deign to step foot on the chain store strip of the Champs-Élysées is to visit the Biologique Recherche spa for seasonal facials. There's no better way to achieve a healthy complexion than through their line of products and customized treatments.

Ambassade de la Beaute, located down a private courtyard, is luxurious, peaceful, and devoted to holistic beauty. Biologique believes there are three stages to healthy skin, which they apply during their appointment. First is the assessment, where they study your skin to develop the most appropriate form of treatment and decide which products are best suited for your skin. Second is initialization, where your skin is cleansed and prepared for rejuvenation by application of their signature P50 lotion. The final stage is application of additional serums and treatment creams to recondition and enhance the skin.

Following a relaxing afternoon of pampering, the Trocadéro woman leaves with a natural, healthy glow.

Biologique Recherche, 32, Avenue des Champs-Élysées

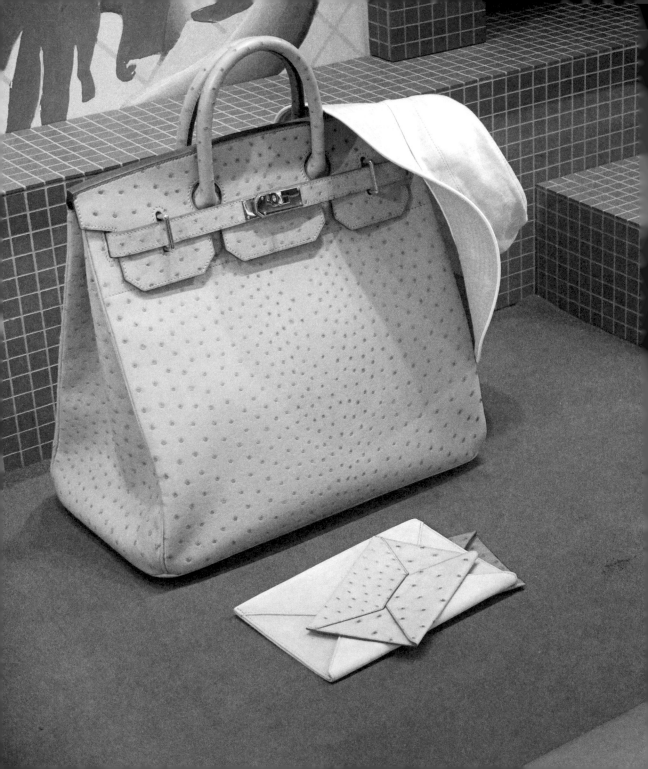

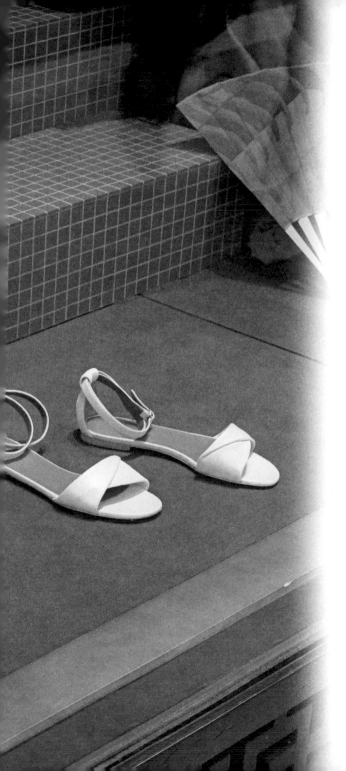

Hermès
24, Rue du Faubourg Saint-Honoré

House of Hermès flagship is four glorious floors of their signature printed silk scarves, Birkin and Kelly handbags, leather cuffs, and even their full line of handmade equestrian saddles and accessories. With a six-year wait and a large price tag, you may not be able to leave with a Birkin bag, but you can still gaze at the beauties on display.

Lanvin
22, Rue du Faubourg Saint-Honoré

Although it's the oldest Parisian fashion house in existence, throughout time, the House of Lanvin has remained true to its modern French chic heritage. Party dresses, fun costume jewelry, classic ballet flats, and embellished sweaters complete the chic Lanvin look by creative director Alber Elbaz.

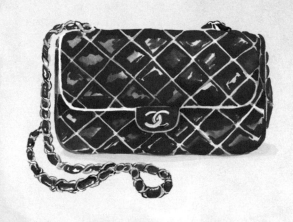

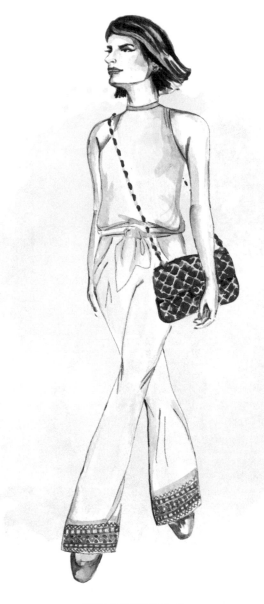

CHAPTER 2
TUILERIES

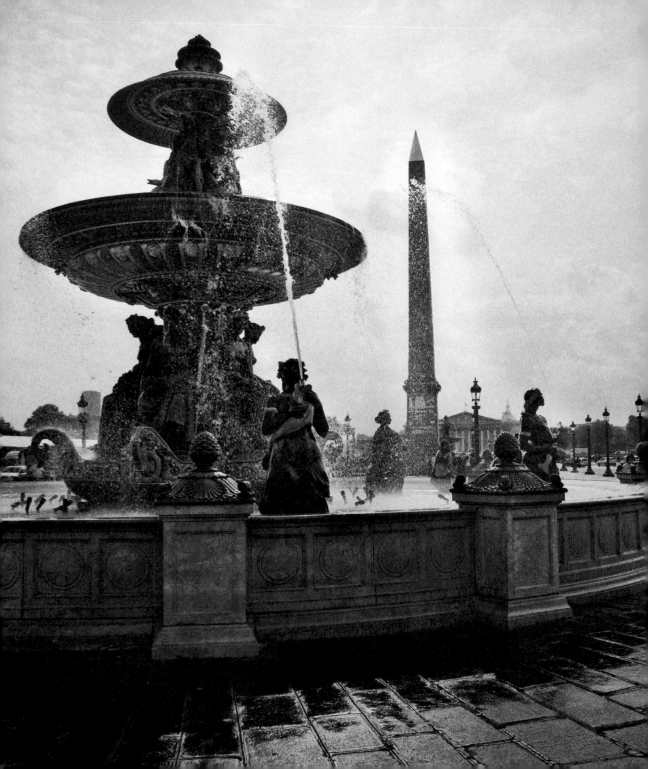

ocated along the river Seine and just east of Trocadéro is the arrondissement known as the Tuileries. When I lived in Paris, each morning on my way to work, I exited the Metro onto the Place de la Concorde—one of the busiest public squares in Paris and main stage for the Tuileries girl. Centered between the start of the Champs-Élysées and end of the rue de Rivoli, the Place de la Concorde is the central connector of the two worlds: the left bank (Rive Gauche) and the right bank (Rive Droite) of Paris.

The centerpiece of this neighborhood is the Jardin des Tuileries, with its perfectly manicured lawns, row upon row of fragrant florals, and one of Paris's only lawns open for picnics. The history of the fashionable Tuileries women dates back to the seventeenth century when the chicest women in Paris roamed the gardens "to be seen." Now you can find them sauntering down the arcades of rue de Rivoli, window-shopping for diamonds in Place Vendôme, or picking up a morning cappuccino at Café Kitsuné in the Palais Royal.

The Tuileries girl may be considered "a Trocadéro woman in training"; her career is on the rise and she aspires to afford regular splurges at Chanel. For now, she's just happy living near the fashion mecca: Chanel's flagship boutique on rue Cambon and, sitting atop it, the former residence of Coco Chanel, with its signature mirrored spiral staircase. Rue Saint-Honoré is her Fifth Avenue, with an array of designer boutiques and the perfect mix of accessory collections like Goyard and Lancaster Paris. The ideal location when she needs a last-minute ensemble for a hot date at the Hotel Costes bar.

The perfect Tuileries morning for a Tuileries girl is spent lounging in the Jardin de Tuileries with a flaky buttery croissant and decadent hot chocolate from world-famous Angelina in hand. This very Parisian breakfast is followed by a stroll through the Musée de l'Orangerie for inspiration from Monet's famous water lily murals. The museum is typically empty in the mornings, allowing her to sit and gaze at Monet's beautiful mix of watercolors in peaceful bliss.

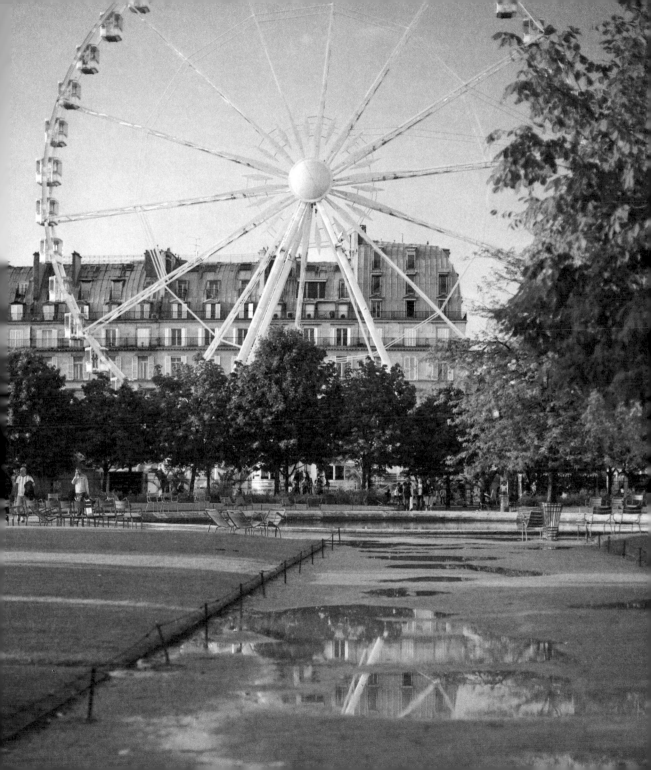

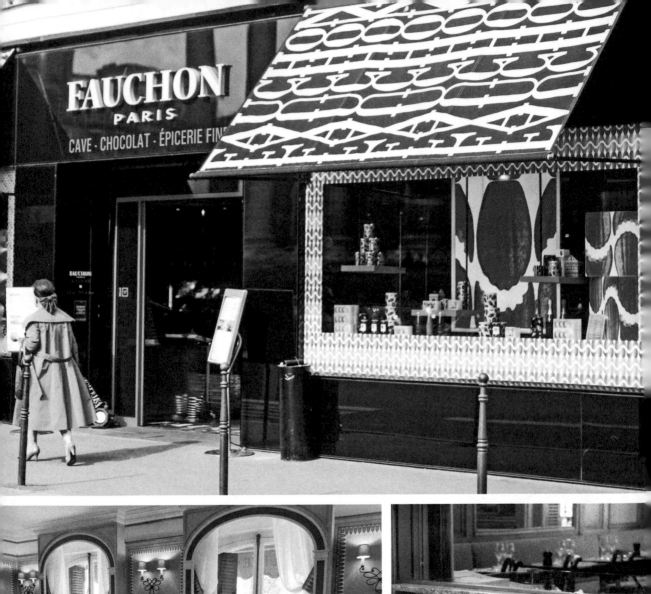
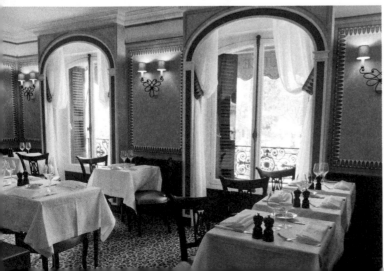
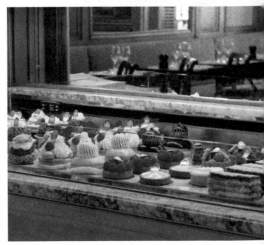

Place de la Concorde

Place de la Concorde is one of the most grand and beautiful squares in Europe. In the 1700s, it was the location of the infamous guillotine that was responsible for the demise of one of my favorite heroines, Marie Antoinette. You may recognize the fountain of gold dolphins and mermen as the one where Anne Hathaway tossed her cell phone after leaving Meryl Streep in *The Devil Wears Prada*. As you pass by, just stop and look for a minute. The grandeur and beauty of its fountains, sculptures, and obelisk center never fail to take my breath away.

Ladurée
16–18, Rue Royale

You'll have pastel dreams in pastry heaven at one of Paris's most special tea salons and restaurants. Stop in for a cup of tea in the late morning or mid-afternoon to spot Tuileries girls enjoying theirs with friends and picking up a few macarons to go. Leave with beautiful candles, specialty macaron items, and a variety of sweet and decadent pastries in Ladurée's iconic mint-green shopping bags. When you get home, decorate your home with the pastel macaron boxes. This sweet memory from your trip can hold makeup brushes, pens and pencils, and more.

Place de la Madeleine

This square is home to a Roman Catholic church that looks more like a Greek temple than a cathedral, a mini flower market, some of the best gourmet shops in Paris, and last but not least, a top-secret address of Parisian women: the chicest public *toilettes* in Paris. Between the flower market and the entrance to the church is a stairway leading to the most beautiful art nouveau–style bathrooms, with intricate mosaic tiling, carved wooden doors, and stained-glass panels. Each stall even has its own period pedestal sink.

Fauchon
24, Place de la Madeleine

Not just the birthplace of Fauchon but also the official birthplace of *Bright Lights Paris*. It was one sunny Parisian afternoon when on a shopping trip with girlfriends that I received the call of a lifetime. I used to think of Fauchon as one of my favorite gourmet shops and must-have opera pastry. Now I'll never forget standing just outside the entrance with my friends Helena, Keiko, and Eliot when my literary agent called, confirming my dreams of writing this book.

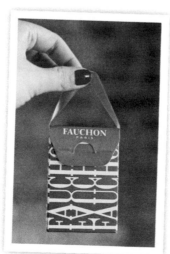

Lancaster Paris
422, Rue Saint-Honoré

I first took notice of the Lancaster Paris handbag collection when seeing their gorgeous ad campaigns in *Vogue Paris*. Shot by one of my favorite photographers, Guy Aroch, the images captured the woman we all aspire to be—chic, confident, and cool. The collection of handbags is a seasonal must-have for Parisians. They are on trend, offer options in the perfect shades of colors and supple leathers, and are also affordable. Whether a bucket bag, satchel, or my favorite, the "Betty Bag" designed by Betty Autier, I carry a Lancaster Paris bag at least a few times a week.

& Other Stories
277, Rue Saint-Honoré

This is a brand started by the H&M Group, so already that screams "cool." Add in blush stamped with a quote from *Romeo and Juliet* and I'm hooked for life. They design a full range of clothing and accessories to mix and match styles. You could leave with a whimsical dress, menswear-inspired oxford shoes, bright-colored mod sunglasses, and even a scented body wash and moisturizer set. Having a personal infatuation with roses, I never leave without a product in the Rose Revival scent.

Chanel
31, Rue Cambon

The flagship boutique, the couture atelier, and the space of Coco Chanel's apartment. The monogrammed awning welcomes you to the world of Chanel, with pristine displays holding pieces made of ethereal silk, classic tweed, and soft quilted leather. Even if you aren't able to purchase a handbag, go in to purchase a Glossimer or fragrance just to walk out with the signature black-and-white shopping bag.

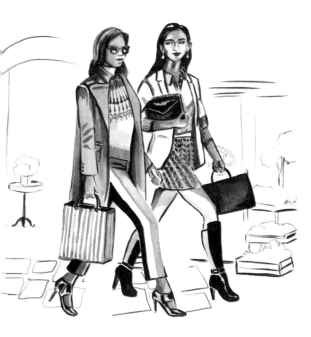

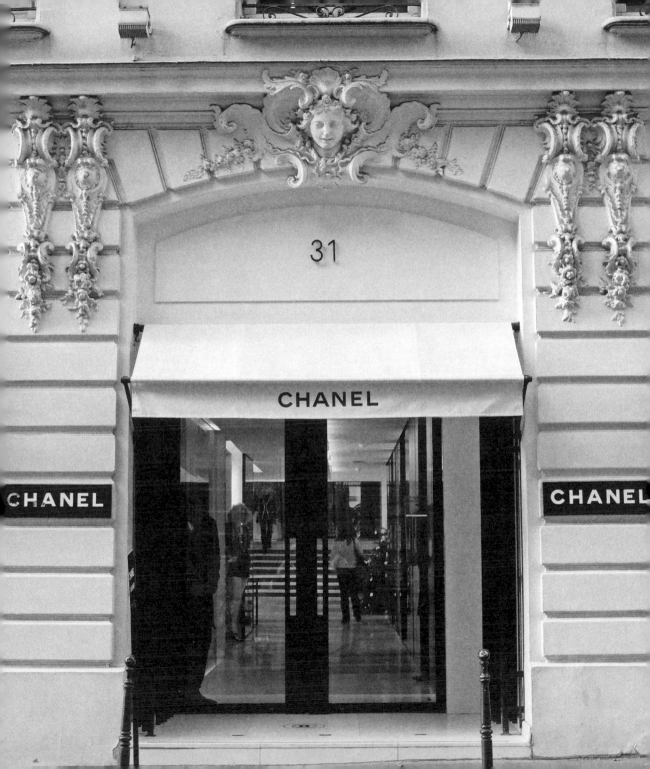

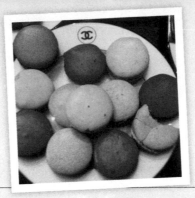

TEA AT COCO'S

Many of my friends work in fashion, and a few lucky ones travel to Paris each season for Fashion Week. It was one July a few years ago I decided to tag along during couture week—not to attend shows, but just to hang out with my girlfriends in Paris. It was a few days before my flight when I received a call I'll never forget. Penny had already arrived and had just left a meeting at Chanel. She called to notify me to pack a special outfit for a very special occasion as we were going to have tea at Coco Chanel's apartment. Tea at Coco's?!? Not just any outfit would do, but it had to be a little black dress. While Coco didn't invent the LBD, she made it a part of fashion history in the 1920s when *Vogue* stated her dress was "a uniform for all women of taste." That sunny Paris afternoon, I wore a black silk Rebecca Taylor dress with lace inset neckline and cap sleeves, with pink Max Mara ballet flats and my navy Chanel handbag. Yes I know, Max Mara is Italian, but if you saw the shoes you'd understand why they were the ideal choice. They are the perfect color pink—not too pastel and not too bright. A shade Coco would have approved of.

From the point we entered the flagship at 31, rue Cambon, each moment was more magical than the last. We walked up the famous mirrored circular staircase and past the couture atelier and offices. Coco's apartment, with Oriental décor, is on the second floor, but she never actually spent the night there and instead used the space to entertain friends and clients. She believed a woman should keep her private life just that . . . private . . . and did so herself by discreetly living in a penthouse room at the Hotel Ritz across the street. Overlooking Place Vendôme, her former suite can still be booked for a very steep price.

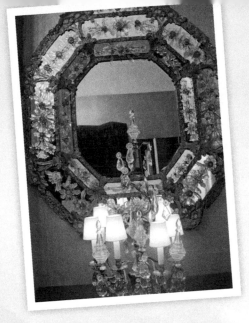

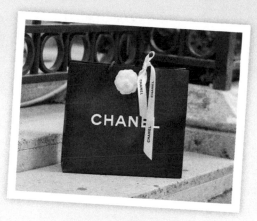

As Penny and I enjoyed our Mariage Frères tea and Pierre Hermé macarons on Chanel-logoed china plates, a Chanel historian shared intricate details about Coco's home décor and trinkets around the apartment. What a pleasure it was to learn so much about a woman I look up to and admire, not just for her style but for her ideals and way of living. It's an experience I will forever cherish, and I'll always be thankful to Penny for sharing such a sweet Parisian moment with me.

Coco Chanel thought of the important needs of independent women when designing her collections. With handbags, she designed very specific pockets to be used in just the right moments. The small outside pocket located on the back of the flap bag was to keep cash so that a woman could quickly and discreetly have access to tip drivers and bell captains. My favorite is the secret pocket inside the bag added to hide love letters she received from a beau.

The House of Chanel has done such an incredible job of capturing her life and most treasured décor items in their current collections, fashion shows, and ad campaigns. From the mini birdcage on her living room side table that inspired Vanessa Paradis's "Coco" perfume campaign in 1992, to the shape of their signature Première watch, which was designed after the shape of Chanel's home on the Place Vendôme, they have been able to keep the spirit of Coco Chanel alive for future generations to experience.

—Arielle Kebbel, ACTRESS

My favorite thing about Paris is the passion that exudes from the people! One of my most epic memories was when I happened to arrive on the night of Nuit Blanche and was told, "It's the one night a year everyone stays up all night!" Museums were open till three or four a.m., and believe me, there were lines at three a.m.! Parisians were in the streets drinking, laughing, and happy to wander free from here to there. To be a part of that freedom was liberating and intoxicating. I love ending my nights with a sexy dinner at Hotel Costes. Yes, it is expensive. But it's worth every cent. Especially if you are lucky enough to be staying the night upstairs.

Pierre Hermé
4, Rue Cambon

My friend and *BelleAboutTown* blogger, Belinda, completely changed how I taste the macarons at Pierre Hermé. She explained to me that they are similar to a perfume, in that they have distinct "notes." As you bite in, you'll notice three distinct flavors—a top note, middle note, and end note flavor. She's not only brilliant but spot-on. This insight has changed every bite I take into these crispy and creamy macarons. On your next trip to Paris, try it for yourself when biting into Hermé's unique flavors, like chocolate and foie gras or passion fruit and rose.

Hotel Costes
239, Rue Saint-Honoré

When a Tuileries girl has a hot date on a Friday night, her location of choice is cocktails at Hotel Costes. Starting the night with a glass of champagne on the terrace, the couple then makes their way into the sexy and dimly lit den with intimate seating areas to cozy up.

La Corte
320, Rue Saint-Honore

Tucked in a courtyard down a cobblestone alley, you'll find Tuileries girls enjoying a homemade Italian meal. The owners will make you feel right at home, as if you've known them since childhood.

Goyard
233 and 352, Rue Saint-Honoré

You can't miss this boutique with its signature logoed trunks stacked outside. The Goyard canvas with patchwork design was created in 1892. The collection has expanded to a full line of travel cases and luggage, handbags, briefcases, and even pet accessories. I'd love to spend an afternoon reading through their client filing cabinet, which keeps notes of every purchase by name including those by Edith Piaf, Coco Chanel, Sarah Bernhardt, the Rockefellers, the Grimaldis, and more.

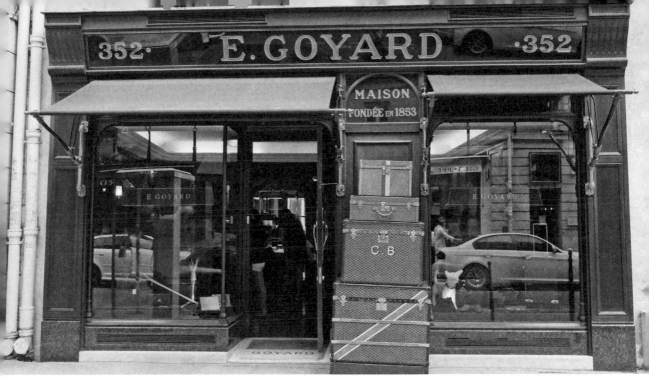

Pierre Barboza
356, Rue Saint-Honoré
————————

This antique jewelry boutique has been open since the 1920s and sells sparkly and pearled treasures dating from the mid-1800s. They also restore old heirloom pieces by adding new stones.

Place Vendôme
————————

A beautiful octagonal shaped "square" with some of the most luxurious and expensive addresses in Paris, home to the history-filled Ritz Paris hotel (if only these walls could talk), town houses, and luxury shopping. Tuileries girls *leche-vitrine* at diamond houses Van Cleef & Arpels, Chanel Joaillerie, Cartier, and Bulgari. Someday she won't just window shop; she'll own a piece in her collection.

The Ritz Paris
15, Place Vendôme
————————

A true Parisian landmark, which just finished a major three-year renovation, this palace hotel is not only where Coco Chanel resided for almost thirty years, but, for a brief time, where George Sand and F. Scott and Zelda Fitzgerald called home. Hemingway used to have his mail sent to the hotel and would read the letters while enjoying his favorite drink—a single malt whiskey—at Bar Hemingway.

Vanessa Bruno
12, Rue des Castiglione
————————

"Laid-back French chic" best describes her collection of silk draped dresses for day and night, oversized cardigans, and trademark totes with sequin trim. It's polished but a little messy all at the same time.

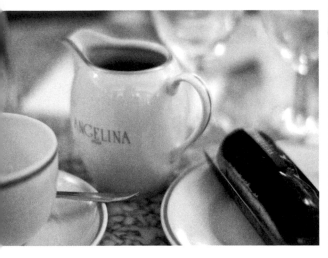

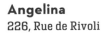

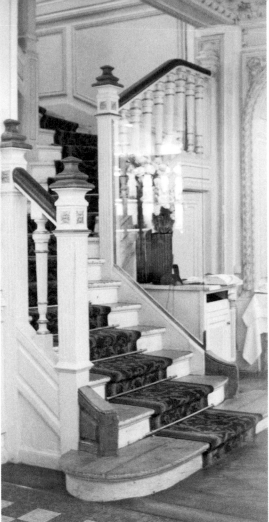

Angelina
226, Rue de Rivoli

Angelina holds the much-deserved title of having Paris's best hot chocolate, and even some would say the world's best. Their signature Chocolate L'Africain is made with four different cocoa beans to create hot chocolate that is thick and creamy, rich in flavor, and has the perfect amount of sweetness. They have a lengthy pastry menu to choose from, and my favorite accompaniment is their equally famous Mont Blanc. It's a heavenly whipped cream concoction on a meringue, which is topped with a sweet chestnut paste piped over the cake. When the lines to sit inside are too long, the Tuileries girl picks up a hot chocolate to go and enjoys it with a stroll through the gardens.

Annick Goutal
14, Rue de Castiglione

The House of Annick Goutal perfumes are inspired by emotion, with the hope of evoking your senses and the ones of those around you each time you spritz. The scents and bottles are feminine, dreamy, and oh so Parisian. One of my favorites is Rose Splendide, reminiscent of a stroll through a garden of roses.

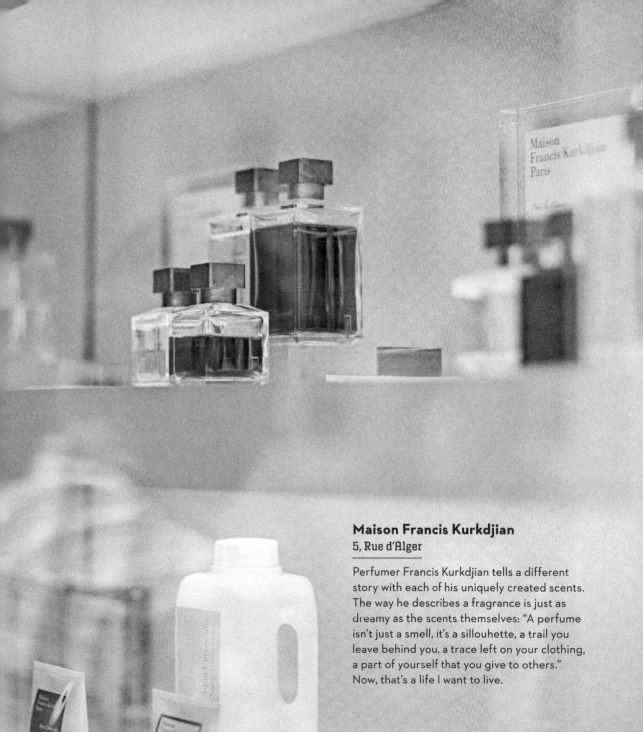

Maison Francis Kurkdjian
5, Rue d'Alger

Perfumer Francis Kurkdjian tells a different
story with each of his uniquely created scents.
The way he describes a fragrance is just as
dreamy as the scents themselves: "A perfume
isn't just a smell, it's a sillouhette, a trail you
leave behind you, a trace left on your clothing,
a part of yourself that you give to others."
Now, that's a life I want to live.

FINDING YOUR SIGNATURE SCENT

The French believe you can tell a lot about a person from their choice of signature scent. I'll admit, spending a lot of money on a fragrance never quite appealed to me. It was rarely an item I even thought about, except maybe in high school, when I couldn't live without a bottle of CK1. That is until my Parisian girlfriends taught me all about the importance of finding your signature fragrance. It's one of the beauty items they splurge on. They believe one's choice of perfume is very personal, and they are even a bit territorial and secretive when it comes to their scents. French women are not keen on sharing their perfume, not even with friends. They prefer to stand out in a unique scent (although they may sometimes spritz on a classic like Chanel N° 5).

At a young age, French girls select their favorite fragrance and are taught how to dab it on their neck, wrists, and never forget, behind the knees. As they get older they learn that a perfume's main purpose is to impress and seduce. A scent can be both delicate and strong and even evoke happy memories of a childhood spent roaming fields of lavender at a grandparent's home or summer vacations by the sea.

When it was time for me to find my signature scent, I was a bit overwhelmed. So I asked my Parisian girlfriends for suggestions on which boutique to visit to help make my selection. The Tuileries girl lives in the mecca of French perfume. Not just the mainstream brands, but almost all of the special niche perfume houses have opened boutiques in her arrondissement. At the top of everyone's list was Annick Goutal for the true Parisian girl fragrance or Maison Francis Kurkdjian for one a bit more daring and truly unique.

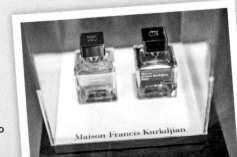

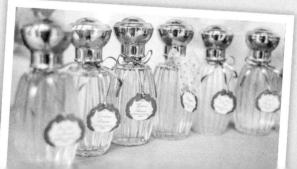

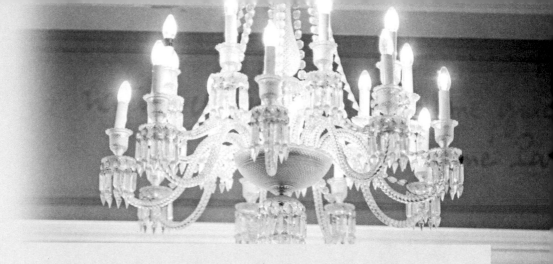

I brought along my boyfriend for an afternoon of scent selecting so we could find something for me and the perfect signature cologne for him. We visited numerous boutiques, and with so many delicious fragrances to choose from, it was a very tough decision. As usual, my Parisian girlfriends were right about the two best being Goutal and Kurkdjian. With completely different scents, they share a commonality in their attention to detail and ability to create a special feeling for their clients. What they create, not only in the scents but also in packaging design and boutiques, is pure perfection.

After collecting many scented cards, we made our final decisions and went back to purchase. His choice of Amyris by Maison Francis Kurkdjian was ideal for him—a mix of woodsy and exotic spices from around the globe. As for me, I couldn't settle on just one and left with a bag from Annick Goutal *and* from Francis Kurkdjian. My choice of fragrance? Well, that's a secret I'll never tell. . . .

Other perfume houses you should visit when in the Tuileries:

Serge Lutens, 142, Galerie de Valois in Palais Royal

Jovoy, 4, Rue de Castiglione

Frederic Malle, 21, Rue Du Mont Thabor

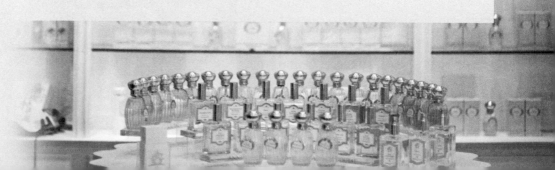

PLACE DU MARCHÉ SAINT-HONORÉ

This quiet square, not far from the hustle of rue Saint-Honoré is full of cafés with outside terraces and a happening Parisian happy hour scene after work.

A few Tuileries girl favorites:

L'ABSINTHE, 24, Place du Marché Saint-Honoré
Affordable bistro of two-Michelin-star chef Michel Rostang.

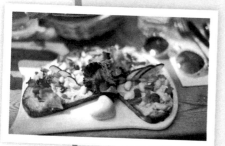

FUXIA, 42, Rue du Marché Saint-Honoré
Incredible salads and pastas. They sell their own bottled olive oil spray and wine.

LE PAIN QUOTIDIEN, 18, Place du Marché Saint-Honoré
Yes, even Tuileries girls go to this Belguim-based bakery and eatery for delicious and healthy food on the go. It's one of my favorites for a quick and healthy breakfast or meal on a Sunday.

Colette
213, Rue Saint-Honoré

One of the first concept shops in the world, Colette is celebrated for their quickly changing window installations, (COACH x Gary Baseman collaboration was a recent favorite) featuring works by world-renowned street artists, and their exclusive lifestyle and fashion collaborations. Pick up chic hats and accessories from Parisian collection Marie Marot, a cool photography book from New Yorker Aaron Stern, and—my dream purchase—diamond bangles by Ofira Jewelz.

L'ecume Saint Honoré
6, Rue du Marché Saint-Honoré

A cute neighborhood oyster shop in the heart of the Tuileries where you can pick up some to go or enjoy a glass of wine with a dozen fresh oysters as they shuck them on the spot.

Astier de Villatte
173, Rue Saint-Honoré

Signature homemade white ceramic dishes and scented candles fill this whimsical boutique like a life-sized curiosity box. Each piece is hand molded and finished in a white glaze showcasing that no two pieces are alike.

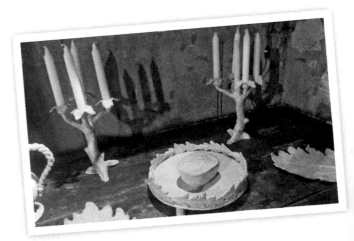

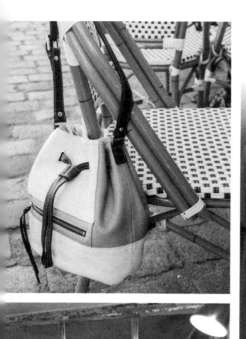

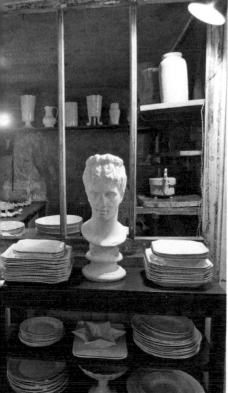

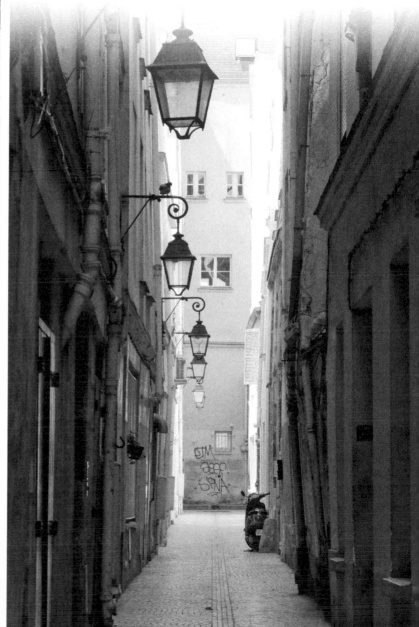

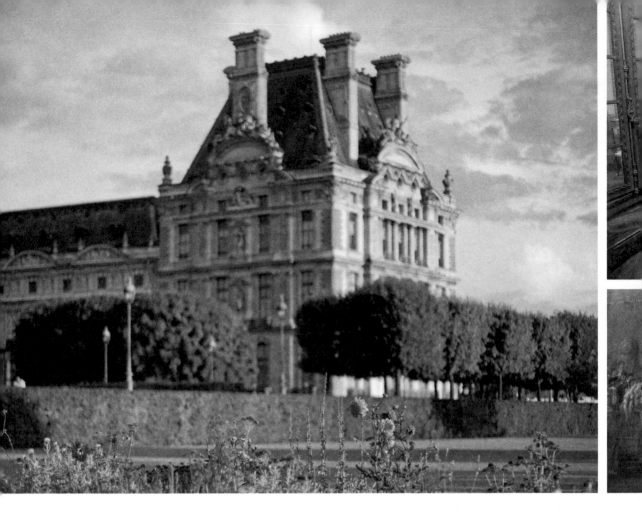

Louvre

I don't think you're allowed to write about Paris without including the Louvre Museum. The former French Royal Palace is incredible, not just for housing thirty-five thousand pieces of art, but for the building itself, which is a work of art that includes the still-intact medievel fortress and royal apartments of Napoléon III. The one thousand security guards are dressed to kill in—what else—suits by Balenciaga. Although a major tourist destination, the Louvre is still frequented by Parisians, who like to wander through on a Sunday morning stroll. A secret tip I learned from a Tuileries girl is how to avoid the long lines at the Pyramid entrance, which can be massive. Instead enter where the Parisians do: directly from the Metro station or the Portes des Lions entrance in the southwest wing of the palace.

Here's a list of my favorite pieces to bring out your feminine spirit:

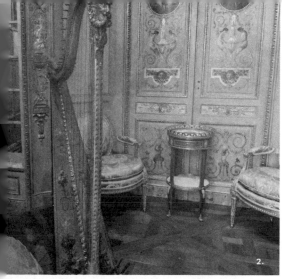

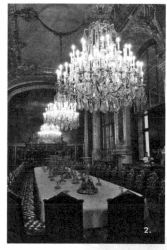

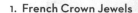

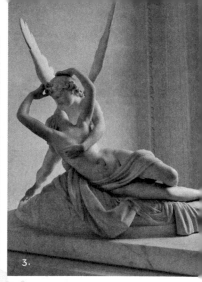

1. French Crown Jewels

2. Royal Apartments of Napoleon III

3. *Psyche Revived by Cupid's Kiss*

4. *The Coronation of Napoleon* by Jacques-Louis David (for Josephine's ensemble)

5. *The Lacemaker* by Vermeer

6. *Diana Leaving Her Bath* by François Boucher

7. *Grande Odalisque* by Jean-Auguste-Dominique Ingres

8. *Madame Récamier* by Jacques-Louis David

9. *Winged Victory of Samothrace*

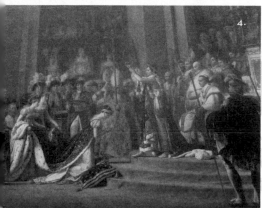

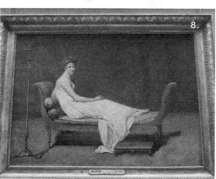

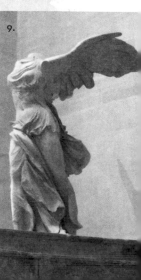

Le Café Marly
93, Rue de Rivoli

One of the chicest outdoor dining experiences in Paris, this café is great for lunch, dinner, or just a glass of champagne. Because it's located under the arcade of the Louvre, you can sit outside rain or shine and experience the grandeur of the palace.

Jardin des Tuileries
Place de la Concorde

Plenty of Parisians occupy this park, enjoying the beautiful flowers, the cafés, and the lounge chairs where they sit to read a book and soak in the sun of Paris. During the winter, an enclosed Ferris wheel takes center stage at the entrance to the park in Place de la Concorde. For summer, a festival of carnival rides and games lines the northern side along Rue de Rivoli.

Musée de l'Orangerie, located in the southwest corner of the Tuileries garden, is home to Monet's breathtaking mural painting, *Les Nymphéas*. Go alone, sit on the bench in the center of the room, and gaze at the paintings. Your view of the water lilies will change when standing close-up and at a distance. The jewel-toned colors of the flowers are magical.

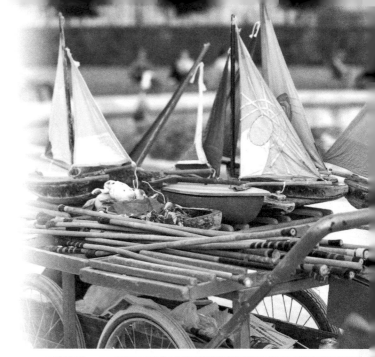

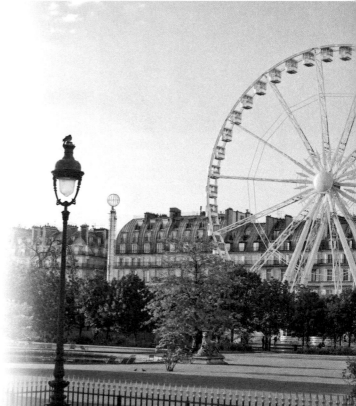

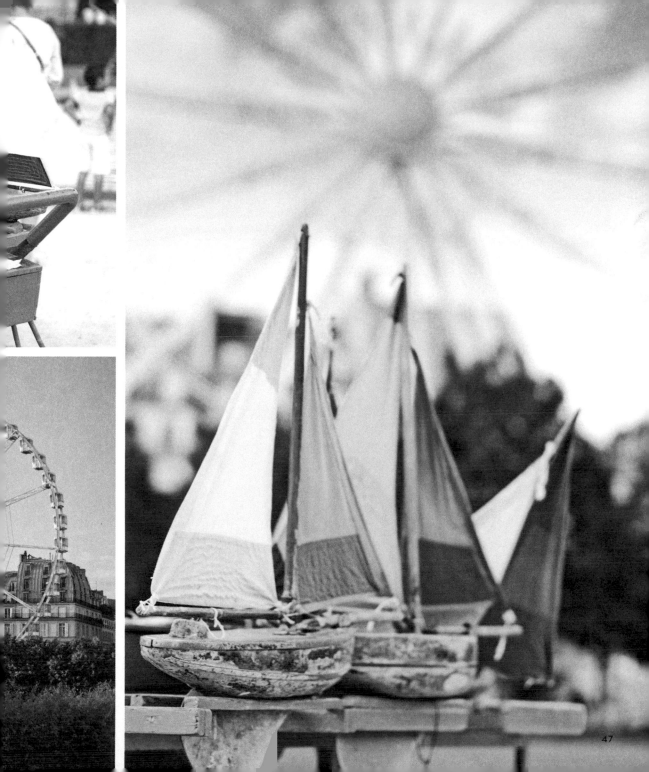

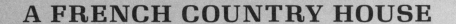

A FRENCH COUNTRY HOUSE

When a Tuileries girl wants to spend a relaxing day out of the city but not travel too far, she rounds up some friends and heads to the Château de Versailles. She loves to picnic on the perfectly manicured French lawn and daydream that they have traveled back in time, discussing jewels and fashion with Marie Antoinette and her ladies at court.

Before leaving her pied-à-terre, she gathers up picnic necessities— corkscrew, canvas tote for groceries, plastic knives and cups, and a sarong to use as a picnic blanket. On their way to the train station, the girls pick up some buttery, flaky croissants for breakfast on the train, and bread, cheese, meat, and a few bottles of crisp Chardonnay for the picnic on the lawn of Versailles. Just like her, you too can prance around the Château de Versailles, rent a boat on the Grand Canal, and paddle yourself to Marie Antoinette's hideaway, the Petit Trianon.

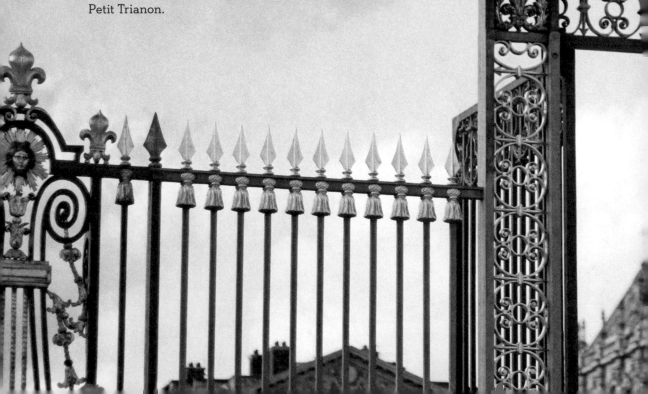

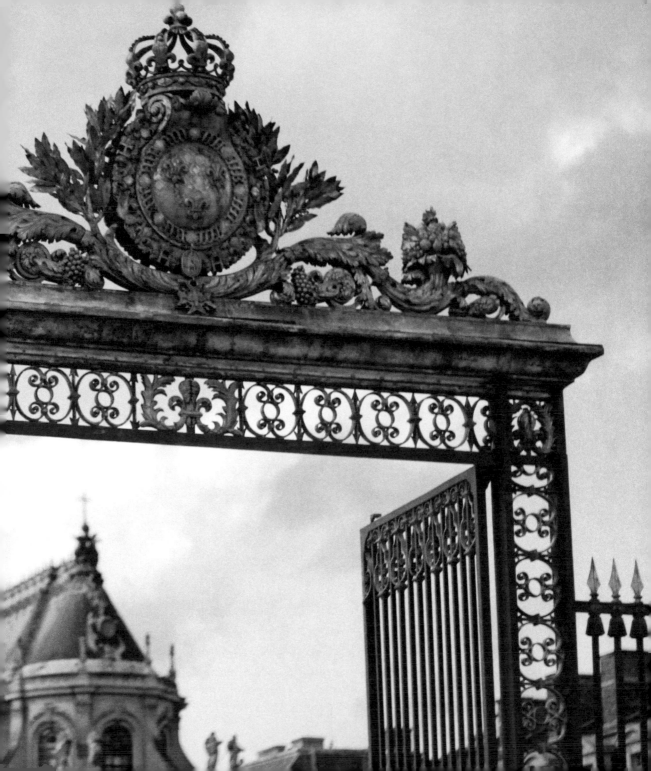

One of the best tips I have learned from my Parisian ladies is to not wear perfume or perfumed lotions on a day you are visiting Versailles. During the warm summer months, the many flowers in bloom there attract many bees, which would also be drawn to the scent of your perfume.

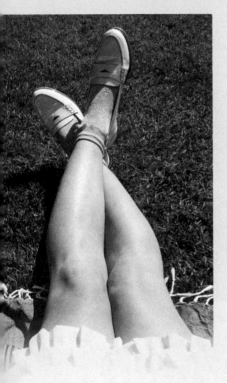

Angelina Tearoom at Château de Versailles

Drink the glorious hot chocolate the way Marie Antoinette would have wanted. Enjoy it in the formal tea salon at the main palace or the more casual café inside the Pavilion d'Orléans. Both are only open to Château ticket holders but absolutely worth it.

The Fountains Night Show

See the Royal Gardens of King Louis IV come to life in this spectacular event. Magical lights and fireworks set to the sounds of a French orchestra illuminate the fountains, which takes place on certain nights from June to September.

Movie Moments

There have been only a few lucky film crews that have been granted access to shoot inside and on the grounds of the Château de Versailles. I'm so jealous of everyone who worked on those films and was able to see, in person, the private halls and rooms once roamed by French royalty.

A Little Romance Diane Lane's first film, made when she was only fourteen, is a sweet story of young love in Paris. In the film, she meets her beau, Daniel, for the first time at Versailles.

Marie Antoinette Sofia Coppola's film starring Kirsten Dunst had exclusive access to certain areas of the château and Marie Antoinette's Petit Trianon. Coppola's film was full of dreaminess, cotton-candy colors, incredible wardrobes, and never too many desserts.

—Georgina Chapman and Keren Craig, **COFOUNDERS OF MARCHESA**

Parisians love one thing more than Paris: leaving town. Take time to go to Versailles and discover "Le Petit Trianon," Marie Antoinette's retreat away from royal duty. It's exquisite eighteenth-century living on a smaller, more intimate scale.

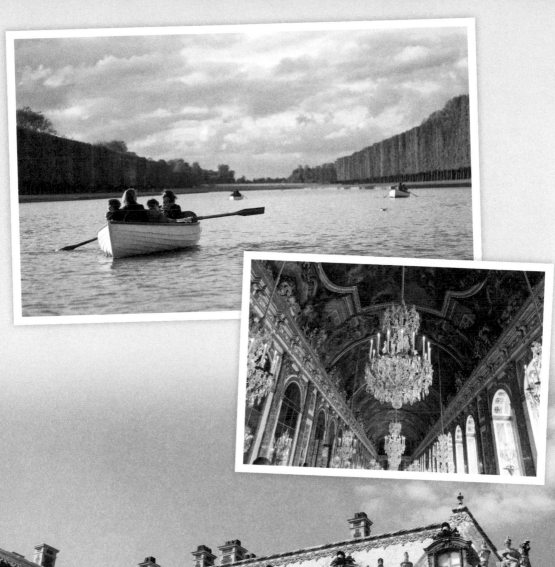
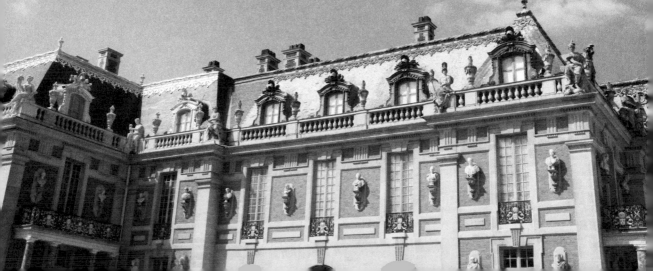

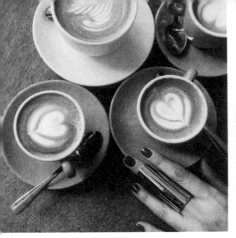

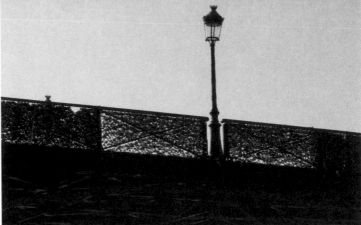

Pont Des Arts Bridge

Located near the Louvre, this pedestrian bridge is a lively spot day and night. Enjoy a sunset picnic with some bohemian Parisians whom you'll find singing and dancing the night away.

Kitsuné
52, Rue de Richelieu

Music meets the fashion world in this boutique that carries the Kitsune collection of traditional pieces with a cool Parisian twist. Kitsuné has continued to be a cult brand in the coolest cities around the world and collaborates with amazing artists and designers.

Verjus Restaurant (and Wine Bar)
52, Rue de Richelieu & 47, Rue de Montpensier

The restaurant upstairs serves market-to-table dishes with a five- or seven-course tasting menu. Downstairs, enjoy small-production wines with a menu of petit plates, which could definitely fill you up for dinner. During the day, Parisians pick up gourmet sandwiches to enjoy in the Palais Royal garden.

Télescope Coffee
5, Rue Villedo

Incredible coffee on a small, quaint street. They don't provide WiFi, so instead you can actually relax and enjoy your coffee without checking your work email or indulging your social media addiction.

Davé
12, Rue de Richelieu

A hole-in-the-wall Chinese restaurant and hideout for the fashion elite. Davé (pronounced Da-vay), is the flamboyant and charming owner who is happy to share some Fashion Week stories of Marc Jacobs's afterparties and nights when Naomi Campbell met up with her pal Lenny Kravitz. Enjoy your meal but note, you definitely dine here for the experience and to meet the restaurant's namesake.

Le Magnifique
25, Rue de Richelieu

Dress to impress at this cocktail bar, and ring the bell to enter. It's one of the few bars in Paris that stays open late. Fashionistas head over around two a.m.

PALAIS ROYAL

The first square built in Paris has a little bit of everything for everyone. Specialty boutique shopping, great coffee, nice restaurants, cafés with outside terraces great for people watching, rose gardens, and even a beautiful fountain. During the weekday you'll spot Parisians at the cafés on their lunch break, and relaxing with a book and picnic on the weekend.

DIDIER LUDOT, 24, Galerie de Montpensier

The most famous vintage boutique in the world. Most known for his vast collection of little black dresses, Ludot has been collecting and selling vintage pieces for more than thirty years. Stop in and be inspired by his exquisite couture collection.

CAFÉ KITSUNÉ, 51, Galerie de Montpensier

Where the cool Tuileries girls go for coffee or when in need of a fresh juice by Bob's Cold Press. Grab a drink to go and enjoy in the Palais Royal gardens.

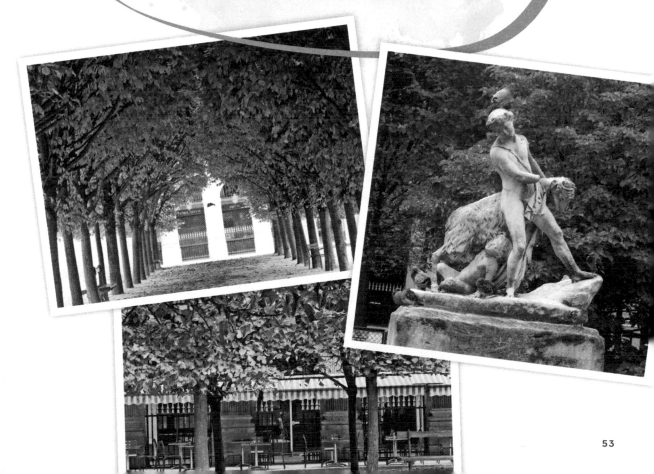

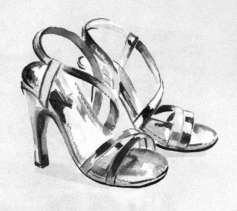

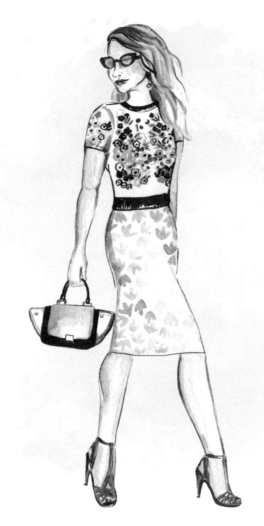

CHAPTER 3
OPERA

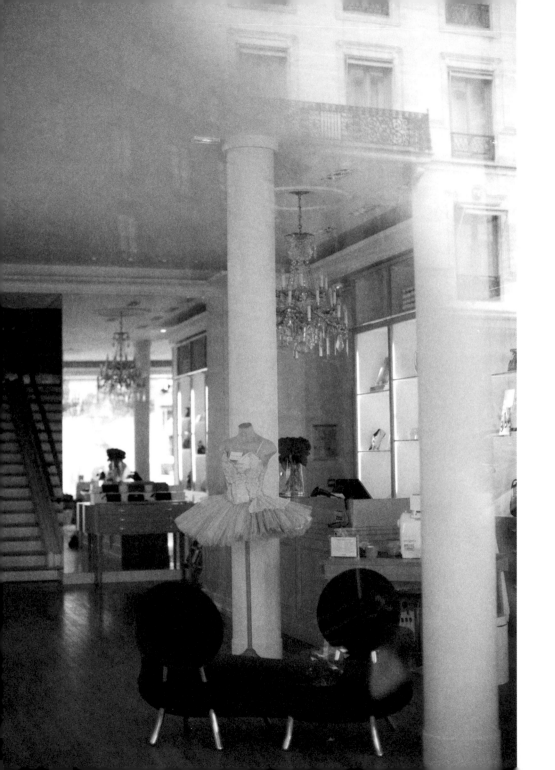

The Opera woman knows how to work hard and play hard. She is a sophisticated and professional woman who elevates her look with stellar accessories. When she's not out at a chic power lunch, you can find her trying on strappy Manolo Blahnik stilettos on the grand boulevard Haussmann, home to two of the most beautiful department stores in the world, Printemps and Galeries Lafayette.

This Parisian knows how to get the most out of her little black dress, taking it from a conservative office during the day to an elegant and chic dinner at night. She is also the consummate shopper, always finding the perfect gift for family and friends at cute boutiques located down Opera's historic passages and narrow shopping arcades.

Some evenings you may find her on a date at the Opera Garnier, for opening night of the newest ballet or opera performance. When summertime arrives, she can be spotted enjoying rosé with girlfriends at the rooftop terrace bar at Printemps. She enjoys cooking at home for her closest friends, and on her way home from work, she picks up some of the best spices in the world at Epices Roellinger. When she's not in the mood to cook dinner on a Sunday evening, she doesn't have to stress about not having restaurants open near her. As luck would have it, she can easily walk over to Little Tokyo on rue Saint-Anne for the best ramen soup and dumplings in Paris.

The Opera woman doesn't live in the trendiest area, but she isn't far from South Pigalle, the burgeoning bobo (bourgeois bohemian) 'hood with new restaurants, bars, and boutiques sprouting up each week. The terrace at Hotel Amour is her pick for weekend brunch, followed by a walk down Rue des Martyrs for fresh fruit and veggies, specialty cheeses, and baguettes from Arnaud Delmontel.

No matter the weather, one place that is always welcoming for girl talk and tea is the indoor garden tearoom at the Musée de la Vie Romantique. The former hangout of Chopin, George Sand, and Delacroix is a quiet spot down a cobblestone lane, where the Opera girl can visit for a relaxing afternoon any time of year.

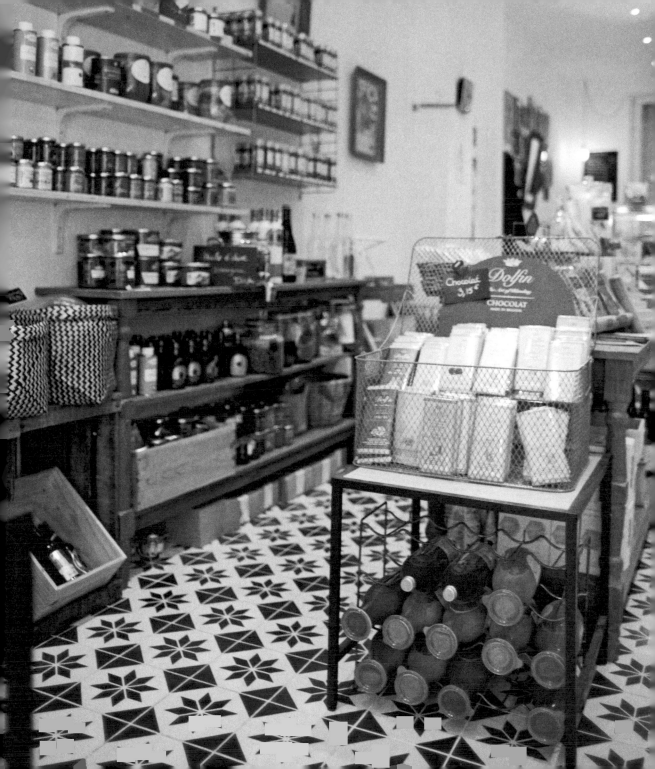

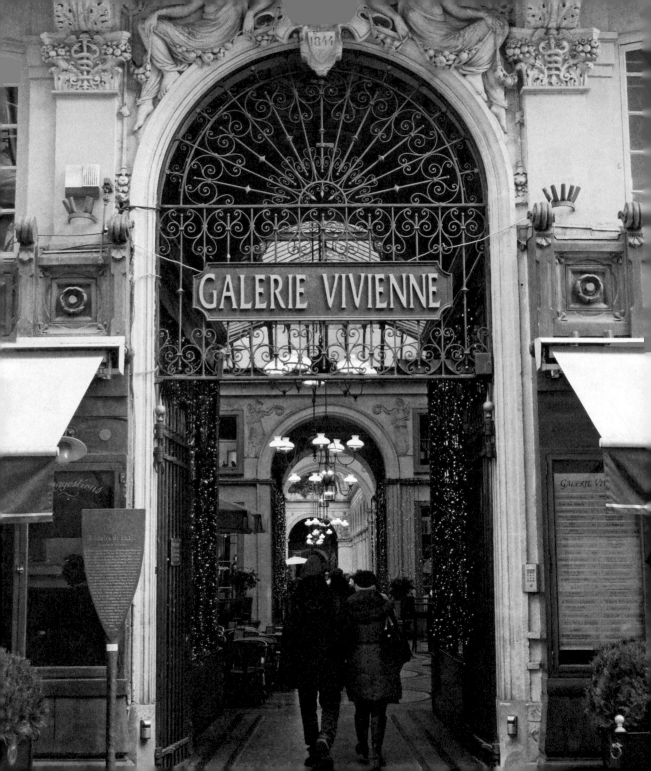

ARCADES

Before there were department stores, Parisian shopping took place at the covered arcades. What used to be more than one hundred arcades throughout Paris is now down to about a dozen, all of which are located on the Right Bank and preserved by the City of Paris. These beautiful covered passageways still contain unique specialty boutiques, cafés, and tea salons. If you get caught in the Paris rain, they are particularly amazing to walk through, or if you just need a break from summer heat or cold winter air. Many still have apartments upstairs with windows that look down on the arcade alleys and Parisians passing through.

GALERIE VIVIENNE, Rue des Petits-Champs and Rue Vivienne
One of the most beautiful of the arcades, with a stunning mosaic tile floor. Stop in for elegant afternoon tea at the lovely A Priori Thé, absorb the creativity of Jean Paul Gaultier's collections in his flagship boutique, and pick up some wine or stay for a glass at one of Paris's most notable wine shops, Legrand Filles et Fils.

La Fontaine Gaillon
Place Gaillon

Actor Gérard Depardieu's restaurant, on a lovely and quiet street, is adorned with a fountain and an outdoor terrace. Specializing in seafood, their seasonal menu is well complemented by an extensive wine list.

Epices Roellinger
51, Rue Saint-Anne

This spice shop from retired three-Michelin-star chef Olivier Roellinger—who is still very involved with his gourmet shop and Maison de Bricourt in Brittany—is filled with spices, vanilla, and vinegars he has found all over the world and the special spice blends that he has created and used in his restaurants for more than thirty years.

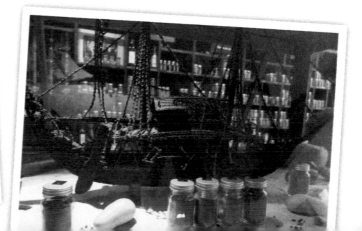

THE MAGIC OF VANILLA

One of my favorite pastimes is baking. It's definitely a skill I learned from my mom, who taught me her secrets to baking the most perfect chocolate chip cookies when I would stay home "sick" from school. Whenever I travel, I love seeking out the specialty baking and cooking shops where the neighborhood women shop. I can find all of the Parisian ladies at the local *épicerie* shops in their neighborhood. I'm probably most jealous of the Opera girls, for they have Epices Roellinger a hop, skip, and a jump away. Opened by retired three-star Michelin chef Olivier Roellinger, it carries Chef Roellinger's specially blended spices—some of the best in the world. He is most famous for his Retour des Indes, a blend of fourteen special spices mixed together to enhance the flavor of certain sauces and meats. His Poudre Grande Caravane is also a favorite of mine and adds an incredible flavor to lamb. Other specialties at Epices Roellinger include cider vinegars, special blends of salt and pepper, and chili powders ranging from 1 to 10 in level of heat.

My favorite section of the entire shop is his vanilla cellar. In a temperature- and light-controlled cellar are preserved twenty strands of grand cru vanilla. To say it's special is an understatement. It's pure magic and opened up a whole new world for me, not just for baking, but also *cooking* with vanilla. The shop has strands from Mexico (the origin of vanilla), Uganda, Tahiti, India, Madagascar, and even the Republic of Congo. I learned which strand was perfect to add to the sauce of a Beef Bourguignon, the one to sauté into a fish sauce or even a vegetable puree. Of course one of my favorites, the New Caledonia strand, has natural crystals that make it sparkle.

Because I was unfamiliar with using vanilla when cooking, Chef Roellinger was kind enough to share some helpful insight. "Use vanilla like you would salt and pepper, to enhance flavors. Once it tastes like vanilla, then you've used too much. Scrape out about a half inch worth for fish, and one inch for beef."

Be sure to stop by on your next trip to Paris and ask for Sandrine. She'll help guide you through their world of spices and vanilla. Once back at home with your spices, you can refer to their website, which gives a great explanation (in English) of the use for each spice and features some of Chef Roellinger's special recipes.

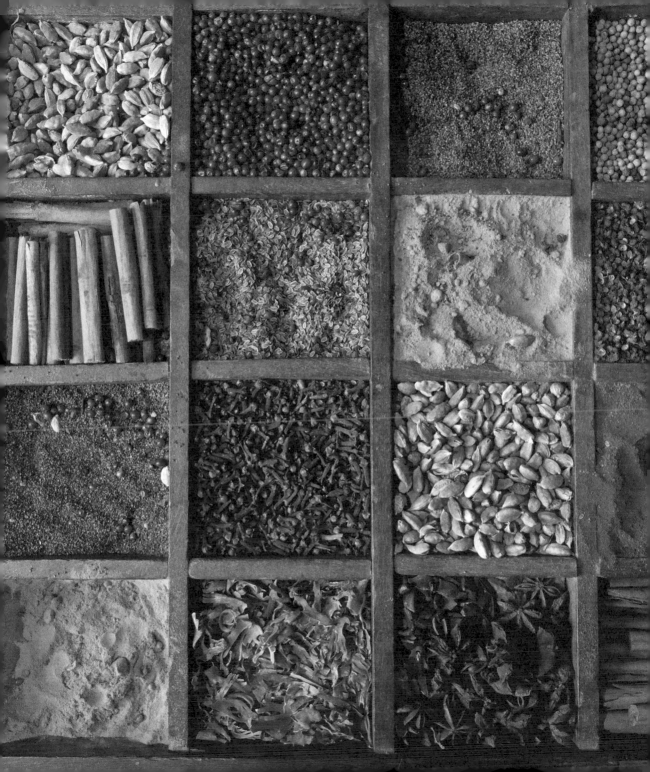

LITTLE TOKYO

Not just full of chic department stores and bistros, this arrondissement is also full of surprises. One minute you've wandered by a grand opera house and the next you've turned a corner to find yourself in Little Tokyo on rue Saint-Anne. This area is a mini village of Japanese restaurants, bakeries, and grocery stores. The tastiest locations usually come with a line of Parisians out the door, but fear not, they move pretty quickly. Ramen and dumplings this tasty and authentic are always worth the wait.

HOKKAIDO, 14, Rue Chabanais
Noodle and ramen bar away from the more hectic area of rue Saint-Anne.

HIGUMA, 32, Rue Saint-Anne
Chinese-style Japanese stir-fry in woks. The gyoza dumplings are so good, go ahead and start with two orders.

NARITAKE, 31, Rue des Petits-Champs
Petite, dive-y noodle bar where the fat-infused ramen broth adds to the already delicious flavors.

Fragonard Parfumerie
9, Rue Scribe

This perfume house was founded in Grasse, a small community on the French Riviera, the world's capital of perfume. But this location is my favorite and includes a perfume museum in a lovely Napoleon III town house. Their mini perfume solids with iconic Paris landmarks on the packaging make wonderful gifts and are easy to travel with.

La Maison du Miel
24, Rue Vignon

The family-run "House of Honey" has supplied Parisians with the best honey in France and beyond since 1905. Saffron or lime honey from France, thyme honey from Spain, and cherry or eucalyptus honey from Italy are just a few selections, along with some from exotic locations such as Tasmania, New Zealand, and Sicily. Learn about the health and beauty benefits and even pick up some soaps and body lotions made with honey.

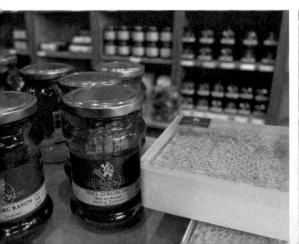

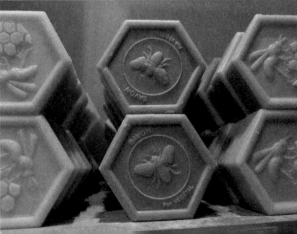

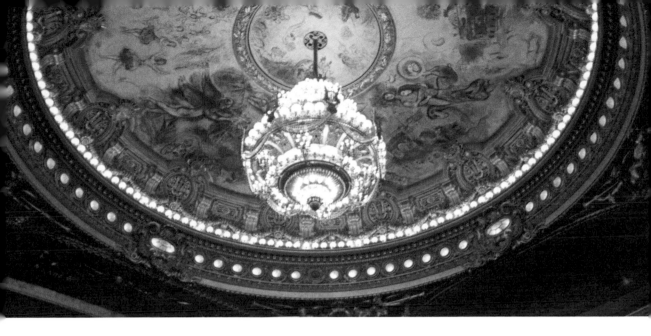

Opera Garnier
Place de l'Opera

Parisian ladies frequent the Opera Garnier to see a ballet, opera, or a night of lovely orchestra concertos. If you think the exterior of this building is lovely, wait until you step inside. Commissioned by Napoléon, the opera house features ornate marble staircases that lead the way upstairs to grand foyers and salons. As you enter the main theater, you'll fall in love with the dreamy jewel-toned mural by "the great artist" Chagall, which is complemented by the bronze and crystal chandelier hanging in the center of the room. By now you may have noticed a theme incorporated into the décor and architectural elements: a lyre. This stringed instrument can be found throughout the building. See how many you can spot in the mosaics, chandeliers, doorknobs, and statues.

—Isabella Boylston, **PRINCIPAL BALLERINA WITH AMERICAN BALLET THEATRE**

The Paris Opera House has tons of history and hidden secrets. I've been lucky enough to take classes there many times and explore the backstage area. There's a room with huge gilded mirrors and frescoes behind the stage where the dancers warm up before the show. There's also a sort of hidden balcony that wraps around the room high up near the ceiling. In centuries past, men of wealth and privilege would sit on the balcony, watch the ballerinas warm up, and send notes down to their favorite girl, inviting her on a date following the performance.

W Paris Hotel
4, Rue Meyerbeer

This nineteenth-century building is the first W Hotel in Paris. (Finally!) The contemporary hotel mixes old and new Parisian styles with art from some of the world's top graffiti artists and illustrators. When she's in the mood for a martini or an old-fashioned with a twist, the Opera woman meets colleagues or friends at Bar Brûlé, with a spectacular view overlooking Palais Garnier. Their restaurant, Coquette, serves delicious dishes 24/7. Save up your Starwood Preferred Guest points and book one of the W's suites from fantastic to fabulous to wow; you can't go wrong.

GRAND SHOPPING

Two of the most prestigious and beautiful department stores in the world happen to be located next to each other on the boulevard Haussmann. If you have only a short time in Paris but need a lot of retail therapy, I recommend you first head to Galeries Lafayette and Printemps. You may spot an Opera woman in one of the shoe salons on her lunch break or picking up a couple of new Chanel Glossimers, but it's largely an international clientele. If you need to refuel mid-shopping, you don't even need to exit the store as they each have more than a dozen eateries and pastry shops. If you're in Paris during the holiday season, stop by to admire the celebrated window displays and glorious Christmas tree inside Galeries Lafayette.

GALERIES LAFAYETTE, 40, Boulevard Haussmann
Here you'll find nine stories of shopping in the main building, with two smaller buildings for home and men's merchandise. This one-hundred-year-old Belle Epoque structure, with a magnificent glass dome ceiling, even dedicates a building across the street to gourmet food, with more than three hundred varieties of cheese, three thousand bottles of wine, and a champagne counter. You can also visit outposts of Angelina, Pierre Hermé, and Le Pain Quotidien.

PRINTEMPS, 64, Boulevard Haussmann
This impressive shop boasts a 7,500-square-foot shoe department with the best selection of designer, contemporary, and less expensive brands. Stop by L'Atelier Repetto to design your own custom pair with choice of 252 colors in lambskin leather, a selection of border and lace colors, and the option of having your initials printed on the inside. A lovely glass cupola sits above Brasserie Printemps to enjoy as you dine, or stop by Cojean for fresh salads. There are three Ladurée bakeshops, and the World Bar, with masculine décor, in the men's store. Toast your new stilettos on the rooftop bar with a glass of rosé wine, overlooking Paris and a stellar view of the Eiffel Tower.

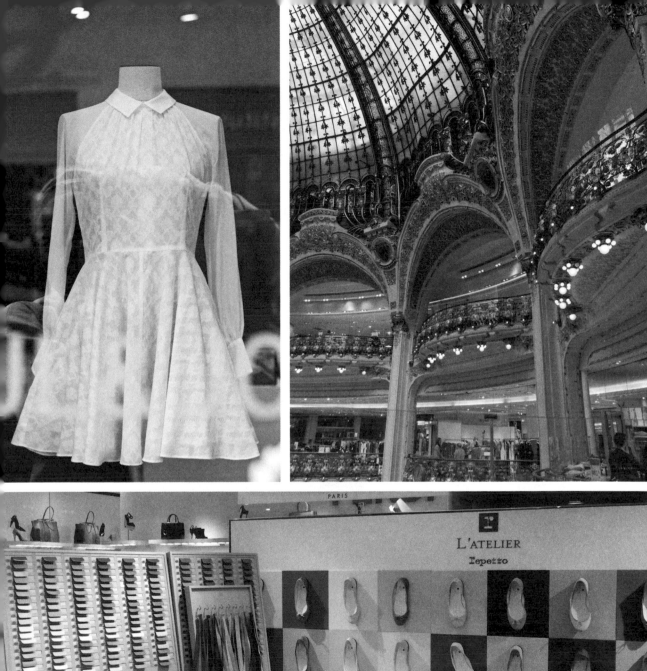

La Conserverie
37, Rue du Sentier

On a side street, this bar and music venue will take you back in time with retro décor and signature cocktails topped with rock candy. You'll find a chic Parisian crowd and a menu of gourmet food in tins—foie gras, sardines from Brittany, smoked salmon, and caviar.

Musée de la Vie Romantique
16, Rue Chaptal

This ivy-covered mansion and cottage-style garden tucked away on a quiet street celebrates the spirit of the Romantic Movement. Previous home of painter Ary Scheffer, who entertained friends such as George Sand, Chopin, and Delacroix, the museum provides a whimsical look at their lives and the romantic world they created. The museum will get you in the mood for love with works by French Romantic artists. Parisian ladies enjoy the lovely garden conservatory tearoom, open from March to October.

Le Carmen
34, Rue Duperré

French composer Bizet's former residence, now a cutting-edge cocktail bar, was named after his famous opera. Le Carmen draws in a rock 'n' roll crowd with its decadent boudoir-themed space and superlative drinks. With no set cocktail menu, the expert barman can create something to suit your mood and favorite flavors and ingredients.

Buvette
28, Rue Henry Monnier

It's rare to hear that a French *gastrotèque* first became a huge success in New York City prior to opening in Paris, but when you try Chef Jody Williams's menu, you will understand. As a New Yorker, I'm spoiled with daily access to her West Village location, but when I'm in Paris I can't help but pop in for a Croque Forestier. Once you have one, I bet you'll share my obsession.

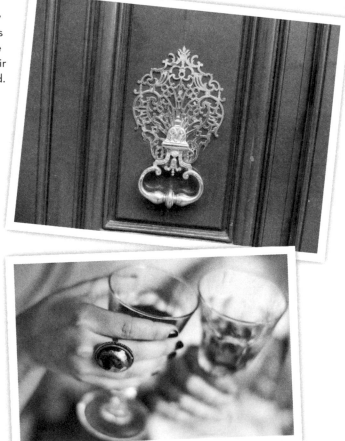

YOUR OWN PARISIAN TERRACE

When I'm walking around Paris, I'm constantly looking up at all of the beauty and intricate details of the historical buildings. One of the features I love most, and one that probably makes me the most jealous of Parisian ladies, is the small balconies so many of the homes have. Many are filled with fresh flowers and herb, but it's the signature table and two chairs that I adore the most. I love to daydream about what it would be like to wake and have morning tea on my own Parisian terrace, or in the evening join my boyfriend for a glass of Pinot Noir and chat about our day.

On occasion I catch a glimpse of a Parisian woman reading her *Vogue Paris* while sipping on morning coffee, or in the evening chatting with girlfriends with a glass of wine and a cigarette. I wonder if they know how lucky they are. The terrace is just part of their everyday life, and I'd settle to have that for a week.

At my home in Brooklyn, I have a small backyard I am lucky to call my own. After returning home from a recent trip to Paris, I purchased an almost identical bistro set on Overstock.com. Of course it's not exactly the same, but every bit of Paris that I can have at home helps me miss it a little less. Whether it's inside your home, in your backyard, or on roof deck, you can create your own Parisian terrace to inspire your inner Parisian girl.

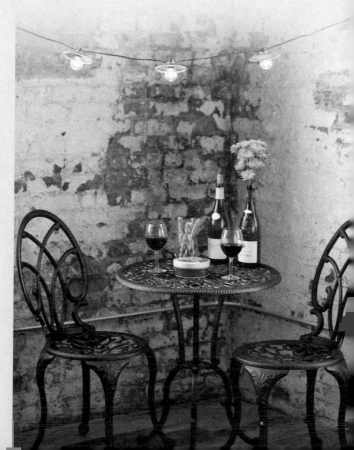

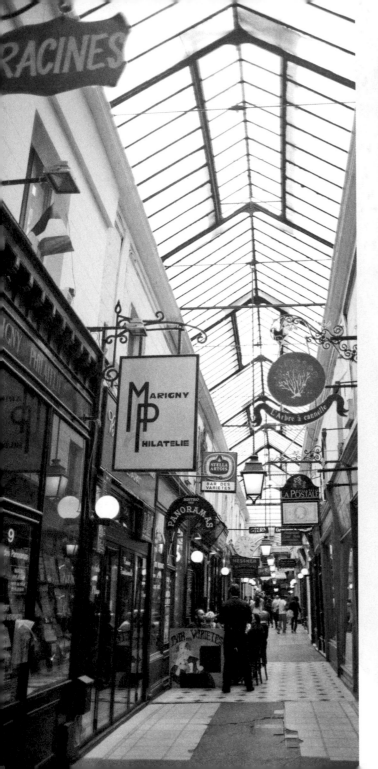

PASSAGE DES PANORAMAS

Paris's oldest covered passageway was once notorious for its courtesans and was the first public space in Paris to install gas lamps, in 1817.

PASSAGE 53

Parisians love this small two-Michelin-star neo-bistro. With no set menu, you have a choice of five or eight dishes. The chef's selections are simple but inventive and revealed course by course. Count on some of the best meat dishes in Paris, as they have a small family perk: the owner's stepfather is Hugo Desnoyer, the most acclaimed butcher in Paris.

GYOZA BAR

It was opened by the team at Passage 53, and you can count on the freshest high-quality ingredients in this twelve-seat dumpling bar.

CARTES POSTALES & LETTRES ANCIENNES

This is a lovely vintage postcard shop. It's so special to read what others used to write to their friends and loved ones. I also love finding postcards marked with significant dates in my life such as a birthday or anniversary.

Two Wine Bars
Where You Can Shop for
Wine and Stay for a Meal

Racines specializes in natural wines with a small but stellar bistro menu. Coinstot Vino serves Brittany oysters and more, with a large selection of wines.

RUE DES MARTYRS

This busy street buzzes with pedestrian traffic as Parisians come for the gourmet food shops; fresh market vegetables, fish, and meats; and sweet bakeries. It's an Opera girl's one stop to buy delicious food and treats for a gourmet picnic with friends. For a Parisian immersion, take a walk on a Sunday morning and shop with the local ladies and gents.

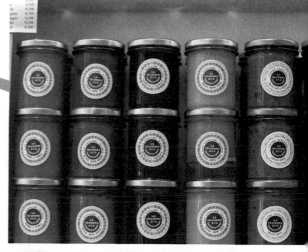

La Chambre aux Confitures, no. 9
Homemade jams and dessert spreads

Premiere Pression Provence, no. 9
Olive oils and vinegars from the South of France

Arnaud Delmontel, no. 39
One of the best baguettes in Paris

Rose Bakery, no. 46
Pick up or stay for fresh organic soups, sandwiches, quiche, and salads

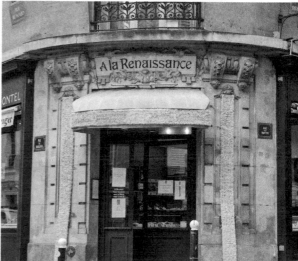

Terra Corsa, no. 42
Their specialty, Corsican cured charcuterie, is epic

Popelini, no. 44
Here, sweet choux à la crème pastries line the counter and are sure to be the next Parisian sweet treat taking over your instagram feed

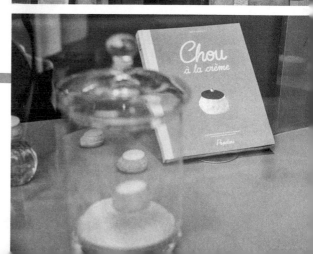

Emmanuelle Zysman
81, Rue des Martyrs

This is the self-taught jewelry designer's flagship boutique and workshop. Featuring beautiful pieces of hammered and chiseled gold that are dainty and feminine, just like Parisians ladies prefer their jewelry.

Mamie Blue
73, Rue de Rochechouart

This three-story vintage store contains an epic collection of clothing and accessories. You may spot one of your favorite French designers shopping here for runway inspiration.

Hotel Amour
8, Rue de Navarin

French graffiti artist André opened this hotel, which gets booked up by fashion photographers, editors, and Brooklyn hipsters. The interior garden terrace fills up with Parisians for weekend brunch.

La Pantruche
3, Rue Victor Massé

An affordable neo-bistro by Chef Franck Baranger, whose menu brings comfort food to another level. The oyster tartare, braised beef cheeks, and for dessert a Grand Marnier soufflé baked to perfection is my idea of the perfect meal.

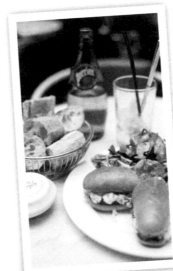

Karine Arabian
4, Rue Papillon

Former accessories designer at Chanel, Karine Arabian designs unique shoes and handbags that are truly special pieces. A little bit 1940s, with opulence and sexiness.

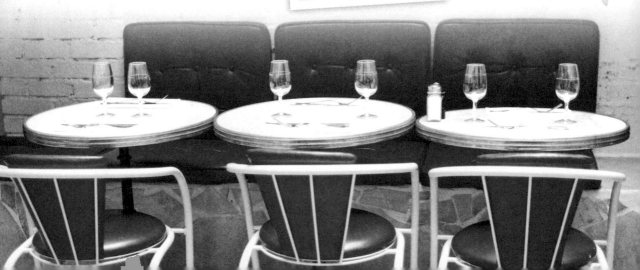

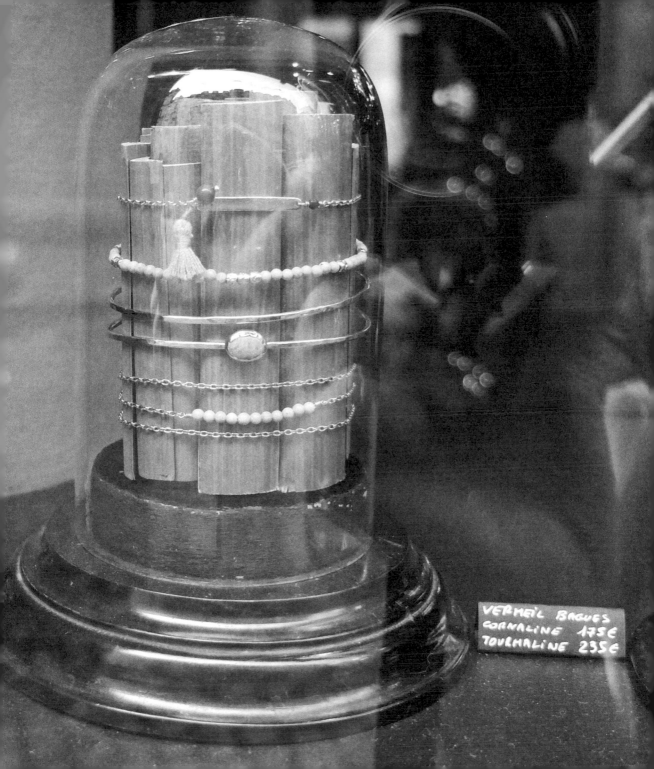

VERMEIL BAGUES
CORNALINE 175€
TOURMALINE 235€

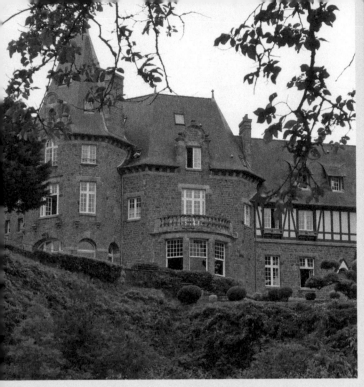
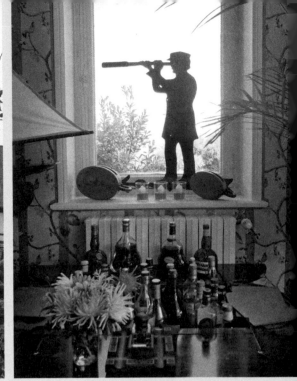
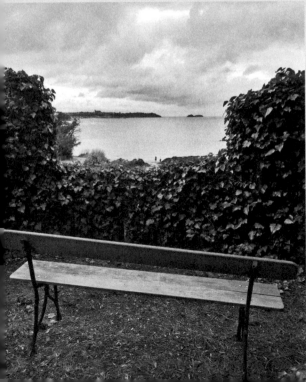
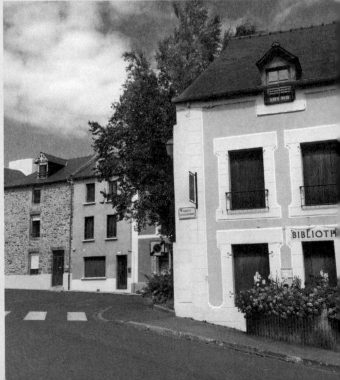

A WEEKEND IN BRITTANY

When my friend Celine wants a weekend escape with her boyfriend, they head to her family's cottage on the Brittany coast. Of course I had to experience what she describes as "a calming and romantic retreat from city life in Paris." Home to quaint seaside villages, baskets of oysters at every sidewalk café, and the famous Brittany stripe shirts, it's the perfect weekend getaway.

With many villages to discover and not sure where to start, a helpful tip from Sandrine at Epices Roellinger helped make our decision quite simple. She suggested we visit and stay at Chef Roellinger's beautiful Château Richeaux near his hometown of Cancale, Brittany. After falling in love with his spice shop in Paris, I couldn't imagine staying anyplace else. From Paris, we traveled the TGV train to Saint-Malo, passing fields of sunflowers and medieval churches in tiny villages. A quick cab ride, courtesy of the animated Italian driver, Gerard, brought us to the Relais & Châteaux hotel, renovated and opened by Olivier and Jane Roellinger.

Château Richeux is a petite and romantic seaside châteaux with luxurious rooms and cozy and serene outdoor seating areas. We happily stayed in a garden-level room, with our own back patio overlooking both the garden and the cliff-side sea view. It was heavenly! In Brittany, the tide of the English Channel goes in and out two times a day and at different times throughout the year. At low tide, we took a romantic stroll along the beach, and in about forty-five minutes we arrived at the quaint sea village of Cancale.

When we first entered the main port, we explored the tiny back alleyways leading to homes and a few bed-and-breakfasts. I fell in love with the lovely window boxes filled with blooming flowers that coordinated with the colorful windows and doors. Next, for lunch, we delighted in a grand mer seafood platter. It was rather adventurous, with some unidentified crustaceans new to my eyes and taste buds, but fun and delicious to try. Exploring the village at the top of the hill was next on the agenda. A quiet area with beautiful stone buildings is home to shops and bakeries, Olivier Roellinger's spice shop, and the prettiest library I have ever seen.

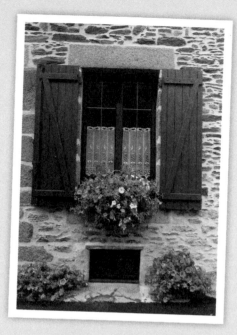

With all the walking and hiking around the village, we took a taxi back to the château and rested up for an incredible dining experience at their restaurant, Le Coquillage.

Our evening began with a glass of Chardonnay and amuse-bouches on the back terrace overlooking the English Channel. While perusing the menu, I realized that there was no need to ask what the "catch of the day" was since the entire menu was made up of what was caught fresh that morning. Chef Roellinger has worked exclusively with the same fishermen and farmers for years. There's one for lobster, crab, and shrimp; one for seabass; one for clams; and one for oysters. He believes that when you're cooking a meal, you're the last part of the story; the story begins with the fisherman in Cancale catching the fresh sea bass and lobsters and the farmer hand-selecting freshly picked carrots and strawberries, while his dairy cows are feeding on salt field grass, enhancing the flavor of their milk. These local purveyors take such care not only selecting the produce, but also transporting it to the chefs they supply. When the restaurant receives their food, the chefs begin their magic, mixing exotic spices, secret ingredients, and sautéing buttery sauces to delight your taste buds.

The following morning we enjoyed a quiet breakfast on the back patio of our room and promised to return again soon, next time for a week, to explore more of the magical villages of Brittany and nearby Normandy. Maybe even go horseback riding up to World Heritage Site Mont Saint-Michel.

Château Richeux /Restaurant Le Coquillage
Le Point du Jour, Cancale 35350 France

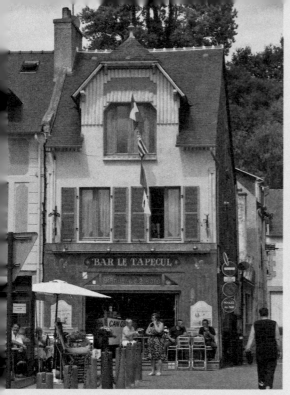

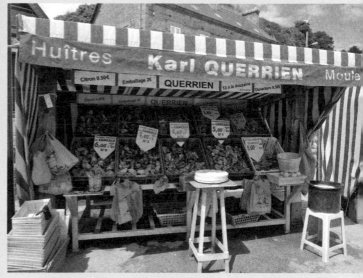

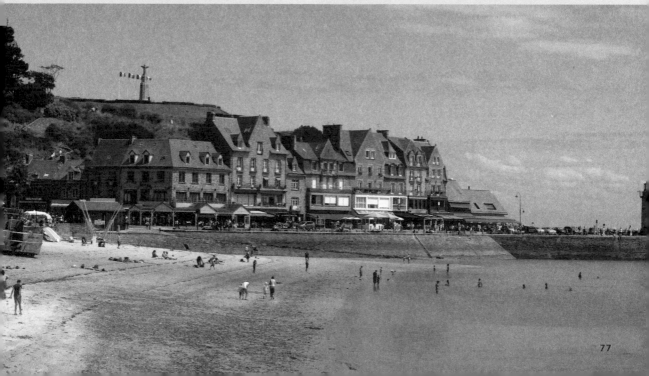

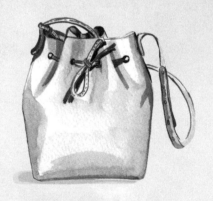

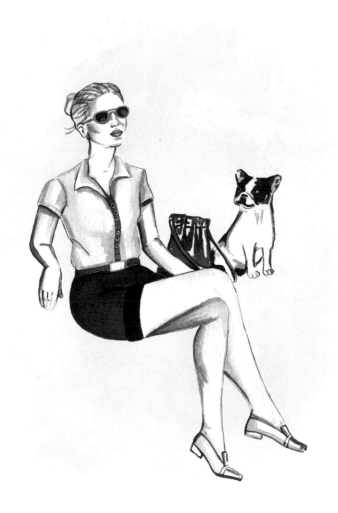

CHAPTER 4
MONTORGUEIL

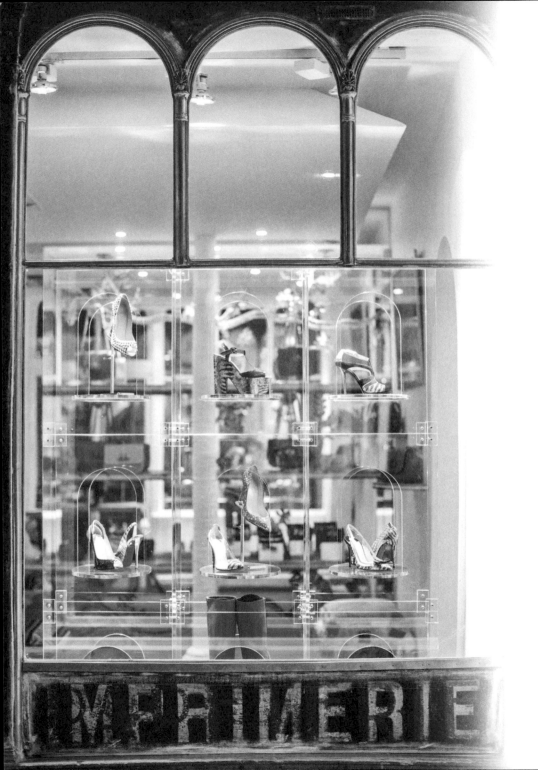

Wandering east from the Tuileries, you'll arrive in Montorgueil, a neighborhood in the heart of the Right Bank with office buildings galore. If you ignore the masses and allow yourself to get lost in the charm of Montorgueil, you will find some of the most quaint streets the city has to offer. It's important in all of your sightseeing that you follow the example of Parisian girls and always find a time and a place to sit down somewhere, anywhere, and simply do nothing. Just be in Paris. One of those quiet streets perfect for that is rue Bailleul, which is home to one of my favorite restaurants in Paris, Spring. I love it not just for the incredible food, but for being full of the most fashionable women in Montorgueil.

The Montorgueil girl is quite the chameleon. She can stand out in bold pieces or keep her look subtle and low-key. She lives near the busiest Metro station in Europe, Châtelet, where she can easily head to Charles de Gaulle Airport and pop over to Greece for a relaxing weekend trip to the beach.

By the way, if you happen to be in Châtelet, or any Metro station in Paris for that matter, take notice of the performers and even stop for a few minutes to enjoy their talents. All of the musicians and singers must audition to perform in the subway stations, and they will delight you by singing and playing their hearts out with the most beautiful music. If you want to hear good music aboveground, head to rue des Lombards for some of the best jazz bars in Paris and some favorite date spots for Montorgueil girls.

In the northern section of Montorgueil is some the best shopping Paris has to offer, with multi-brand boutiques carrying collections you will never find in the U.S., and a block full of "Frenchies" (café, wine bar, and restaurant). On weekends, you'll spot the neighborhood ladies on rue Montorgueil, a must-visit market street with some delectable food shopping and relaxing cafés. Immerse yourself among them and in a bowl of buttery mussels and frites.

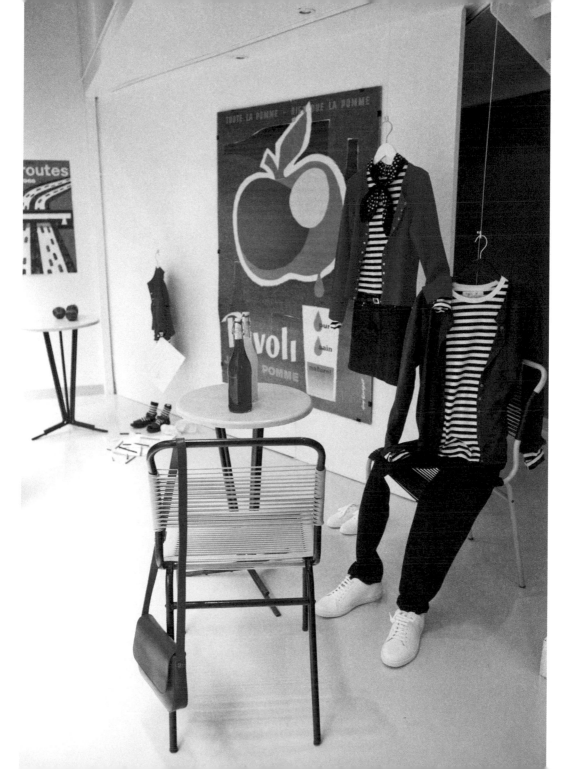

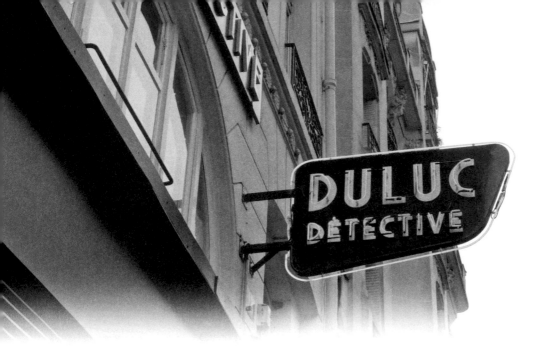

Le Fumoir
6, Rue de l'Amiral de Coligny

Yes the rumors are true: a non-tourist destination just a few blocks from the Louvre really does exist. Here you'll find stylish Parisians enjoying an after-work martini or dinner, magazine editors meeting for lunch, or a hip couple canoodling in a dark corner in the downstairs Library Bar. Enjoy your meal on the terrace during warmer months.

Le Garde Robe
41, Rue De l'Arbre Sec

The assortment at this neighborhood bar a vin includes mostly natural wines available by the glass or bottle. You can order a plate of charcuterie and cheese or a fresh vegetable platter. If you don't finish your bottle, they'll let you take it with you so nothing goes to waste. You can also purchase bottles to go and enjoy along the river Seine.

Spring Restaurant
6, Rue Bailleul

Bring your appetite and sense of adventure to this amazing restaurant, as the only menu you will see is the wine list. Be sure to ask the sommelier for wine suggestions, as he has been voted the best in France. Chicago-born Chef Daniel Rose creates his dishes based on the freshest ingredients available each day at the market. Montorgueil girls love dining here for special occasions.

Duluc Detective Agency
18, Rue du Louvre

If you're in love with the film *Midnight in Paris* like I am, you'll be happy to know the Duluc Detective Agency is available for any of your sleuthing needs. So if you need help tracking down the gorgeous Parisian man you kissed by the Seine the night before, you know where to go.

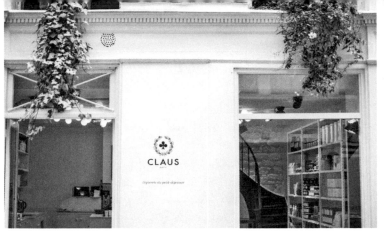

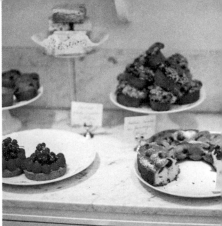

Yam'Tcha
121, Rue Saint-Honore

The name of this restaurant means "drink tea" in Mandarin, and you will certainly want to while enjoying the French-Asian cuisine at this upscale spot. Chef Adeline Grattard works elegantly in her tiny open kitchen while her Cantonese tea sommelier husband delivers tiny cup after tiny cup of perfectly matched teas that pair lusciously with her dishes. The four-course discovery menu is a must-have experience.

Claus
14, Rue Jean-Jacques Rousseau

Specializing in gourmet breakfast, this is the stomping ground for the fashion elite, and not just during Fashion Week. On the first floor, you can get a coffee, fresh juice, homemade granola, pastries, honey, and jam to go. If you're in the mood for a relaxing breakfast or lunch, then head upstairs to their chic dining room.

—Betty Autier, FOUNDER OF LEBLOGDEBETTY.COM

I live in the 2nd arrondissement in Paris, close to rue Montorgueil. Here, you can find everything—restaurants, bars, boutiques, markets, and movie theaters. Claus is by far my favorite restaurant for breakfast and lunch. Everything is organic, fresh, and delicious. My little guilty pleasure is the Apple Bavarois (to share with someone or gobble it up solo if you are starving). What's more, this area is the center of Paris, and that makes each place quickly reachable! I'm just a few steps away from the Marais, a ten-minute walk from the Opera quarter or the rue Saint-Honoré! It's perfect!

THE MAGICAL SHOEMAKER

When I lived in Paris, working as an intern at a fashion buying office, I saved up my money for one fashion splurge. There was no question; I knew it had to be a pair of shoes. I asked my Parisian girlfriends and all of the ladies I worked with where I should go for the most special Parisian pair. Although at that time these two words were a little unfamiliar to me, it was unanimous that I must go to Christian Louboutin. This was pre-*Sex and the City* and before his red soles became the iconic style symbol they are today.

One Saturday afternoon, I met up with my Montorgueil girls for lunch followed by "the moment" I bought my first pair of Louboutins. His boutique on rue Jean-Jacques Rousseau was petite and as special as the unique stiletto heels, pointy ballet flats, and striped espadrilles on display. Following a group vote with the girls, I selected his first edition one-of-a-kind "trash" heels. The pair is more like a museum piece you take off the shelf to enjoy on the days you need that extraspecial touch for an outfit, whether jeans and a tee or a little black dress. Under the translucent top layer is a mishmash of items—a flattened used cigarette butt with red lipstick stain, a feather, part of the boutique address handwritten on a scrap of paper, a used French stamp, fabric trim, and, my favorite, a piece from a strip of 35mm film negative.

Since that day, I have been lucky enough to own a few more pairs and even get to know Mr. Louboutin himself. Not just a magical shoemaker—as my best friend has named him—but he's a magical man. So full of life and happiness, his playful spirit comes through in his designs and collections season after season. His own personal style is so fabulous and accessorized so flawlessly it deserves its own book.

Since my first visit to the boutique, the world of Louboutin has grown into an empire with the addition of a handbag collection, men's shoes, and beauty. Staying true to the history of the brand, his boutique is still open in the Galerie du Passage. The only difference now is it has expanded in size. So while tourists line up to shop at the boutique on rue Faubourg Saint-Honoré, Parisian ladies still shop at the flagship and sometimes catch a glimpse of the magical shoemaker walking through his favorite *galerie* in Paris.

Christian Louboutin, 19, Rue Jean-Jacques Rousseau

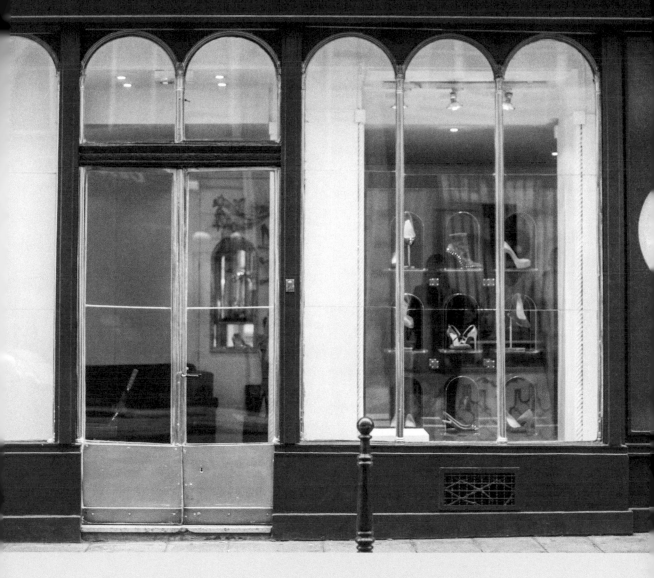

Les Fines Gueules
43, Rue Croix des Petits-Champs

A bistro loved by fashionistas and bankers, Les Fines Gueules is where Montorgueil girls meet their boyfriends for a glass of wine after work and, when in the mood, stay for dinner. The burrata appetizer is a personal favorite, and their meat dishes, from famous butcher Hugo Desnoyer, are always delicious.

Place des Victoires

Historic mansions surround this square, with a monument of King Louis XIV on horseback resting in the center. By day, the square is bustling with patrons visiting the numerous designer boutiques, and by night it is perfectly lit and quietly breathtaking.

Chez Georges
1, Rue du Mail

Julia Child's beloved bistro when living in Paris still looks the same and boasts the same menu, with the most delicious French bistro classics. Duck breast with crispy potatoes cooked in the duck fat is a must.

Lina's
50, Rue Etienne Marcel

When Montorgueil girls need to meet their girlfriends for a quick lunch where gossip and boy talk is the focus, they stop into Lina's. It's a no-fuss spot where you can eat in their café or take it to go. Pick up premade sandwiches, design your own on a variety of fresh breads, or enjoy a fresh salad. While not a classic French pastry, their brownies are so soft and chocolatey, you can't leave without one.

IKKS
5, Rue d'Argout

The IKKS collection is glam rock with modern and feminine pieces to complete your Montorgueil-girl look. Shop for leather bomber jackets, silk floral blouses with tie collars, lambskin leather satchels, and motorcycle boots. While you're there, pick up a great piece for the man in your life.

Mora
13, Rue Montmartre

Pastry chefs from all over the world visit this boutique for the best selection of cake and tart molds, chocolate molds of all shapes and sizes, and other specialty baking accessories.

Zadig et Voltaire
11, Rue Montmartre

Both a men's and a women's boutique, side by side, it offers urban chic collections infused with a casual rock 'n' roll style. One of my favorite brands for supple leather handbags and accessories.

Princesse tam.tam
5, Rue Montmartre

Flirty and fun French lingerie and swimwear collection at great prices. It's one of my favorite boutiques to shop in when I'm in Paris, and I'm thrilled that it is now available in the U.S. You can find it at most Bloomingdale's stores and online at Shopbop.com.

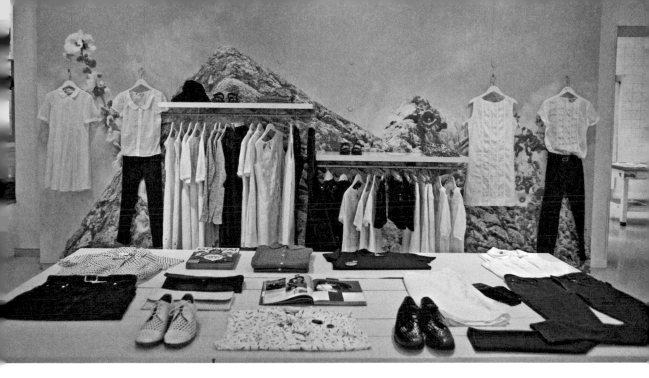

Agnès B.
2, 3, and 6 Rue du Jour

You can't get more timeless French than Agnès B. One-stop shopping to build the perfect Parisian wardrobe, from striped boatneck tops, crisp white button-downs, khaki trench coats, and cardigans in every color. At this largest of all their locations in Paris, you'll find the Agnès B. women's, men's, kids, and travel collections all within reach of the lovely courtyard.

Fifi Chachnil
68, Rue Jean-Jacques Rousseau

Walk through a tiny courtyard to this retro lingerie boutique and behold glamorous styles inspired by 1950s pinup girls. You'll feel girly and feminine and won't leave without at least one matching set.

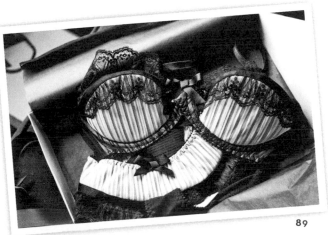

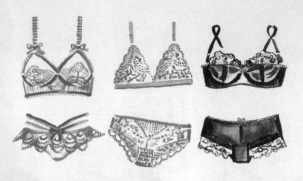

LOVELY LINGERIE

French women celebrate femininity starting with their lingerie. They learn at an early age that the right lingerie wardrobe is as important as owning the perfect little black dress. Parisian department stores even have entire floors devoted to the category, in all price ranges.

The most important rule: everything must match, from your bra and panty sets to what you sleep in. Matching bra and panty sets are not just for special occasions; French women wear them every day. And you should too.

Why all the fuss about lingerie? French women wear beautiful lingerie for themselves as much as for the men in their lives. They feel a certain happiness when wearing something so lovely close to their skin, even if no one is going to see it.

This even applies to sleepwear, which means T-shirts and boxers are a big faux pas. Instead they sleep in silk nightgowns or romantic matching sets.

French women buy bras that accentuate their curves no matter their size, and won't tease men with "faux" cup sizes. Don't shy away from lace or scalloped edges; practical bras don't have to be boring.

For undies, they wear an array of styles from thong to bikini to boy shorts. One of my Parisian girlfriends once told me she buys two and sometimes three different style panties to match one bra to ensure always having a matching set. Pretty genius!

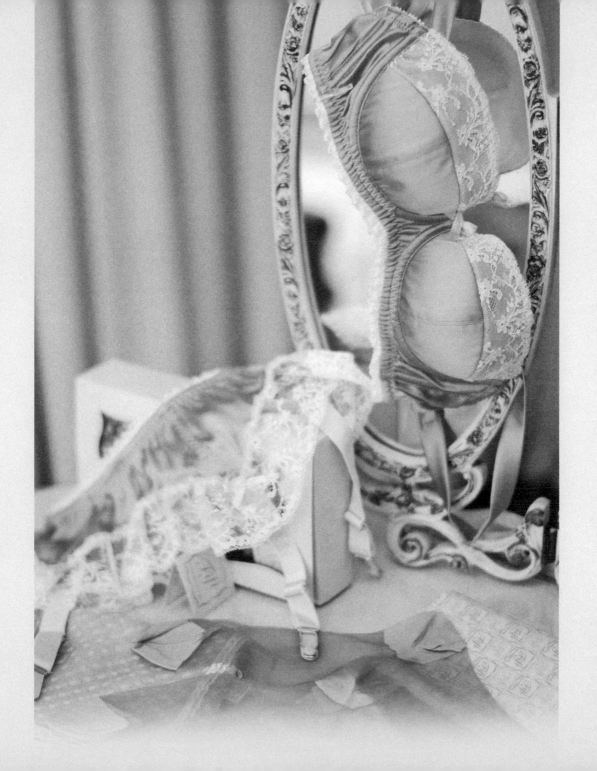

Espace Kiliwatch
64, Rue Tiquetonne

This concept store with a unique mix of new collections and handpicked vintage items is a popular spot. Montorgueil girls stop by almost weekly to see what has just arrived. Pick up cool men's and women's clothing and accessories, limited-edition sunglass styles, and a fashion or design book in their bookshop.

G. Detou
58, Rue Tiquetonne

Floor-to-ceiling shelves are neatly stocked with hundreds of ingredients to bake whatever your sweet tooth craves. This baking-supply shop also carries French gourmet specialties.

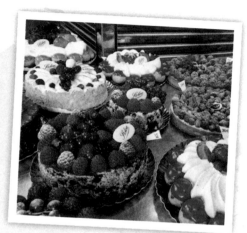

RUE MONTORGUEIL

With one of the best food markets in Paris and plenty of cafés to choose from, this three-block pedestrian street can delight your appetite day and night. You'll find an array of sweet and savory treats along the way.

Here are a few of my "must-taste" favorites:

STOHRER, no. 51
Founded in 1730, this bit of history is the oldest patisserie shop in Paris. They even invented the Baba au Rhum, a delicious rum-soaked pastry.

POISSONNERIE SOGUISA, no. 72
A bustling fish market where chefs and residents get their catch of the day.

AU ROCHER DE CANCALE, no. 78
The last piece of Montorgueil's old oyster market. The menu has expanded beyond shellfish to include salads and tasty burgers. In the winter you can still people watch at an upstairs table right by the window.

BISTRO LES PETITS CARREAUX, 17, Rue des Petits Carreaux
After you've eaten your way through rue Montorgueil, walk toward the end of the block to relax at this low-key bistro. In good weather, take a seat outside on the terrace and enjoy a glass of wine. If you still have room for food, the duck confit and fried potatoes are pure perfection.

L'ATELIER DU CHOCOLATE, no. 45
Their chocolate bouquets and Chokaria, a square block of chocolate layered with caramel and roasted cocoa nibs, make unique, sweet gifts.

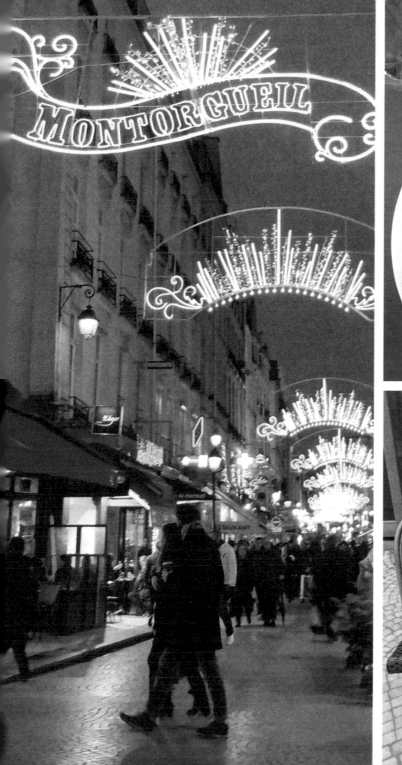
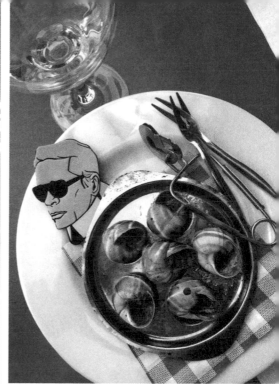
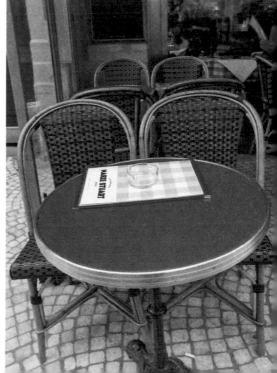

WINE O! WINE

If you ever attend a dinner party in Paris, you may notice that unlike in the U.S., other guests don't arrive with wine for the hosts. The reason is that a French hostess takes special care and thought pairing her meal with the perfect selection of wine. Her local wine shop experts will even ask to know all of the ingredients in her meal to help her select the perfect pairings.

One of my favorite locations to wine and dine and improve my knowledge of French wine is O Chateau. Their wine list, comprised of forty selections, changes each week and varies in price to accommodate all budgets. It includes almost all French wines, with a couple from other countries thrown in the mix.

O Chateau isn't just a restaurant and wine bar, but also a place where the wine brings people together. Here you may notice Parisian girlfriends meeting up after work, a couple on their weekly Friday-night date, and maybe some London ladies in town for a weekend bachelorette party, all with one thing in common—they enjoy and appreciate great wine.

For years, O Chateau has been hosting the best wine tastings in Paris, including lunch and dinner tastings and wine and cheese pairings. Located in a beautiful medieval wine cellar, it's also a great location for private dinner parties and small special events. Parisian girls and visitors to Paris book O Chateau's sunset champagne cruise on the river Seine to celebrate a special occasion or just enjoy some bubbly on a small private tour of the river.

Around the corner from the *cave a vin* is O Chateau's newest venture, Les Caves du Louvre. This former residence of Trudon—who was Louis XV's sommelier—is now a wine-making workshop where, with the help of O Chateau experts, you will learn to blend your own wine, design the label, and leave with a case of your own blend to bring home with you.

I think making wine in the former cellar of the king's private wine collection is about as good as it gets! Soon I'll be returning home with my very own Bright Lights Paris customized blend.

O Chateau, 68, Rue Jean-Jacques Rousseau

Les Caves du Louvre, 52, rue de l'Arbre Sec

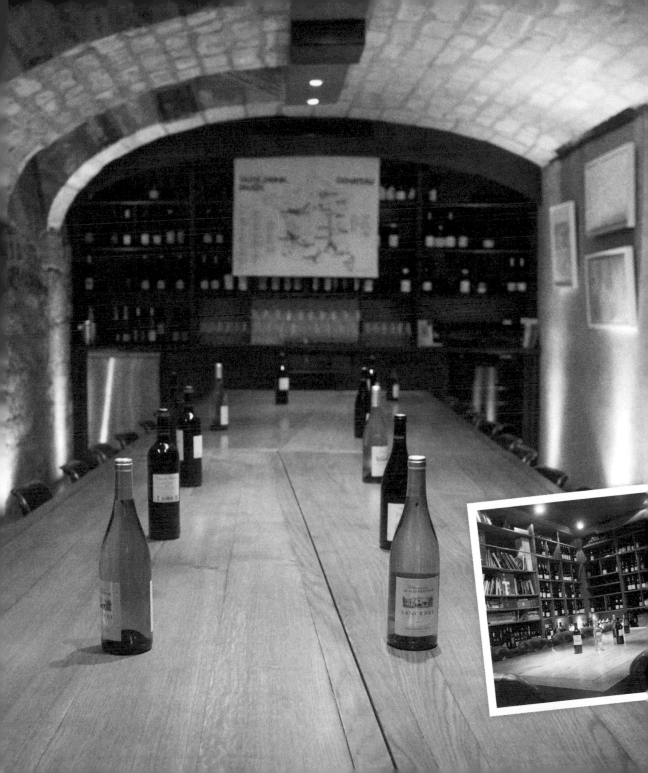

What's wine without cheese? Around the corner from my apartment in Brooklyn is an amazing cheese and gourmet food shop, Stinky Bklyn. I find myself there probably once a week picking up some Comté or Cambembert with slices of fresh prosciutto and gourmet crackers. They are the local experts on cheese and are always helpful when I need suggestions on wine pairings. When entertaining at home or at a picnic, Parisian girls make sure to have the perfect cheese to go with their wine selection.

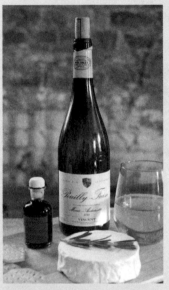

« Pouilly-Fuissé + Cambembert: This raw cow's milk cheese from Normandy has a subtle salty taste with a fruity tang and pairs well with the sweet white wine from Burgundy.

» Chardonnay + Comté Rodolphe le Meunier: Aged raw cow's milk cheese from the Loire Valley, with notes of butter, dried apricots, nuts, and cream matches this full-bodied Burgundy white wine.

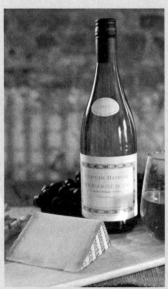

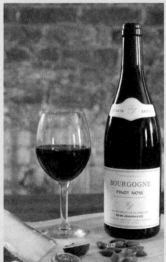

« Pinot Noir + Ossau-Iraty: Raw sheep's milk cheese from Basque Country that is sweet, nutty, and buttery, with notes of hazelnut is best enjoyed with this red.

» Châteauneuf-du-Pape + Pont l'Evêque: Dating back to the twelfth century, this is a pasteurized cow's milk cheese from Normandy. The oniony mushroom flavor is brought out by this full-bodied red wine.

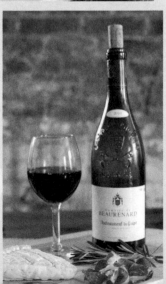

OH, THE FRENCHIES

Chef Gregory Marchand has created quite a delicious block for dining on the tiny cobblestone Rue du Nil. What first started as an amazing restaurant has now expanded to include a wine bar and gourmet breakfast and lunch epicerie.

FRENCHIE, 5, Rue du Nil
No signature dishes due to the daily menu changes, but instead Chef Marchand focuses on signature techniques at his sixteen-seat restaurant, such as smoking fish and meats to perfection and melding different textures of food to enhance flavors of a dish.

FRENCHIE BAR A VIN, 6, Rue du Nil
Wine and tapas bar where you can enjoy a glass while you wait for your table across the street or when you are just in the mood for a light bite with friends.

FRENCHIE TO GO, 9, Rue Du Nil
Petite coffee shop and eatery where all ingredients are made fresh—even their homemade maple-syrup-and-salt-rubbed bacon. Enjoy an egg sandwich or granola and yogurt for breakfast or an assortment of savory sandwiches for lunch.

Experimental Cocktail Club
37, Rue Saint-Sauveur

The first speakeasy in Paris and ranked one of the best bars in the world. Tucked away in a narrow pedestrian street, this hotspot is where Montorgueil girls start their night. My favorite cocktail is their signature Experience 1. It's refreshing, with an exotic mix of lemongrass-infused gin, basil, elderflower, and lemon.

Jefrey's
14, Rue Saint-Sauveur

This cocktail bar has delicious club sandwiches and petit fours to share. Relax on the purple velvet Chesterfield couches, with jazz and soul music playing in the background. Create your very own bespoke DIY martini by selecting ingredients on a printed menu.

Twinkie
167, Rue Saint-Denis

Sometimes the best cure for a bad hangover is a delicious breakfast, but the splitting headache keeps you from deciding what you're in the mood to eat. Devoted to all kinds of breakfast—French, American, English, Mediterranean, and even gluten-free—Twinkie solves the dilemma with savory food and delicious fresh juices. Montorgueil girls also love the kitschy décor of nostalgic childhood toys and games.

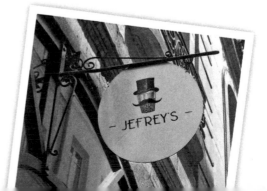

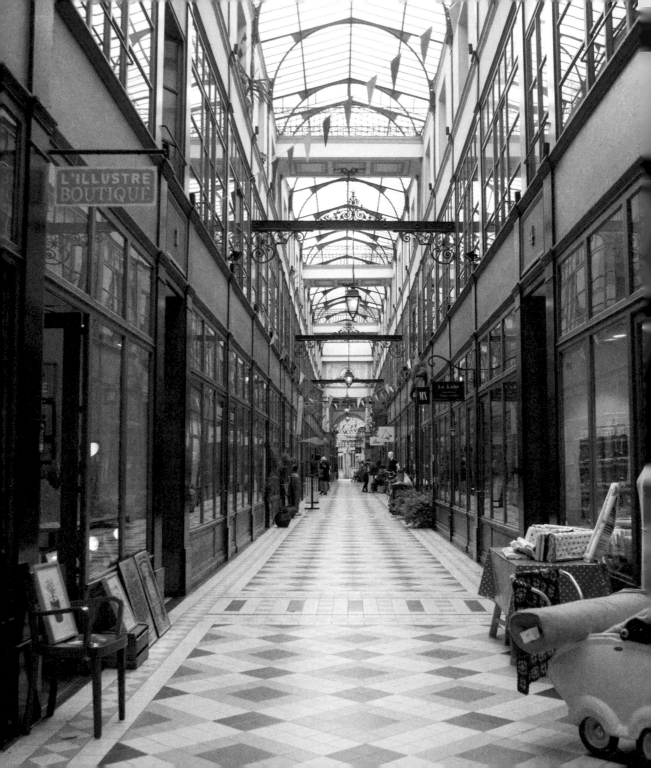

PASSAGE DU GRAND-CERF

145, Rue Saint-Denis

This lovely Belle Epoque passage, built in the 1830s, is filled with small design shops:

L'ILLUSTRE BOUTIQUE, no. 1
Stationery, paper goods, and small pieces of art.

LA CORBEILLE, no. 5
Vintage home décor finds from the 1950s to present.

CÉCILE BOCCARA, no. 8
Cécile designs sweet and whimsical jewelry including dainty headpieces perfect for a Montorgueil girl's special night.

POUR VOS BEAUX YEUX, no. 10
Carries more than one thousand vintage eyeglass frames. Owner Charles Mosa opened his first shop in Nice more than twenty years ago. Frames from the 1930s start at 50 euro and go up to 600 euro.

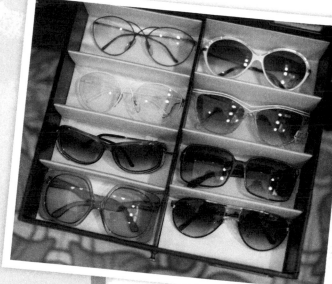

Artist Squat
59, Rue de Rivoli

See what life is like for real Parisian artists by wandering around a true artist squat. In 2006, the building was given to a group of artists by the City of Paris. The installations on the outside of the building change, so always remember to look up in between shoe shopping on rue de Rivoli.

SEASONAL SHOES

When Montorgueil girls want to go shopping for on-trend, inexpensive, and good-quality shoes, they head to rue de Rivoli. Save your money to splurge on classic styles at Christian Louboutin and head here for seasonal favorites that will last a season or two.

ERAM, no. 98
MINELLI, no. 96
HEYRAUD, no. 90

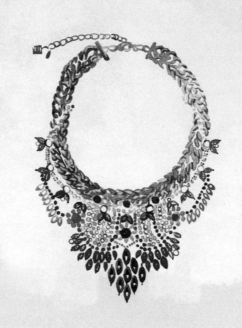

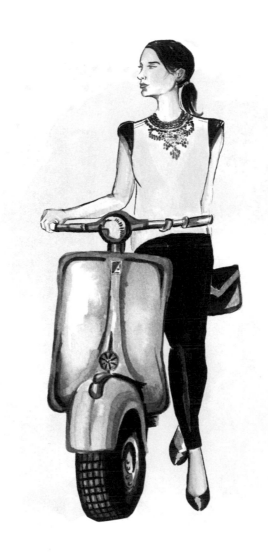

CHAPTER 5

LOWER MARAIS

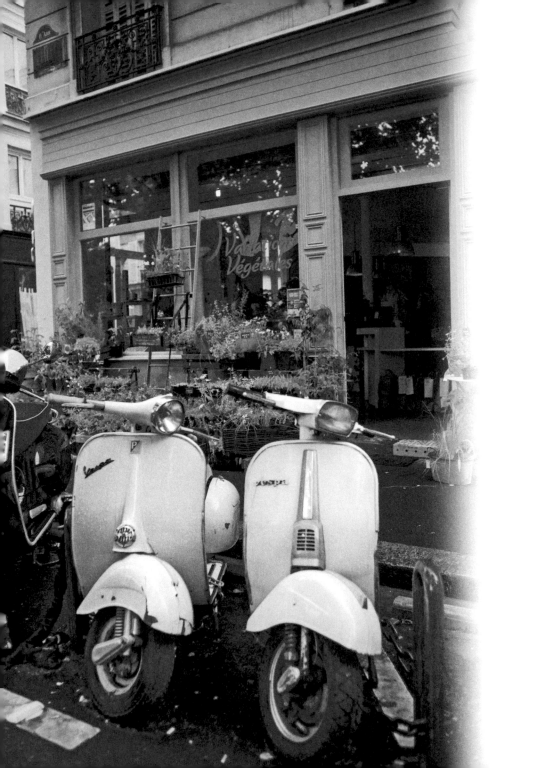

Welcome to the Lower Marais, where I once felt at home for a dreamy and delicious six months. It definitely holds a special place in my heart and still remains one of my favorite neighborhoods in Paris. The Lower Marais woman is a unique kind of Parisian, all her own—and she owns it. She is the definition of effortless chic. In her signature Converse sneakers and motorcycle jacket, she spends her weekend enjoying brunch and shopping with friends. She skips new hot spots for local haunts that have been open for a hundred years yet remain some of the coolest locations in Paris. You can spot her near the Place des Vosges by her trademark accessory—a vintage turquoise Vespa.

Just like the ladies who call this area home, the Lower Marais is eclectic and spicy, with the tastiest falafels, savory crepes, chic karaoke, and the sweetest of pastries. Wandering through some of the oldest medieval streets in Paris, you'll find the best mix of boutiques, from young Parisian designers not found in the U.S. (yes, not even New York City), to sophisticated staples, the best vintage shops, and what I refer to as "The Golden Triangle of the Marais." On the two blocks of rue Vieille du Temple, south of rue des Francs-Bourgeois, you'll find boutiques from the most sought-after contemporary French brands: Sandro, Maje, and Iro. With pieces from those three collections, you'll become a Lower Marais girl in no time.

A great perk of the Marais occurs on Sunday. When most of Paris is sound asleep, its boutiques, bakeries, and restaurants are all open and bursting with energy. During warm months, you'll find outdoor tables at all the cafés packed with the coolest Lower Marais girls. Easy to spot by their tousled hair and simple and clean makeup that highlights all of their best features, they continue to make me wonder how they can have that "just rolled out of bed look" but still be as stunning and fresh as can be. They are the coolest girls in town without even trying.

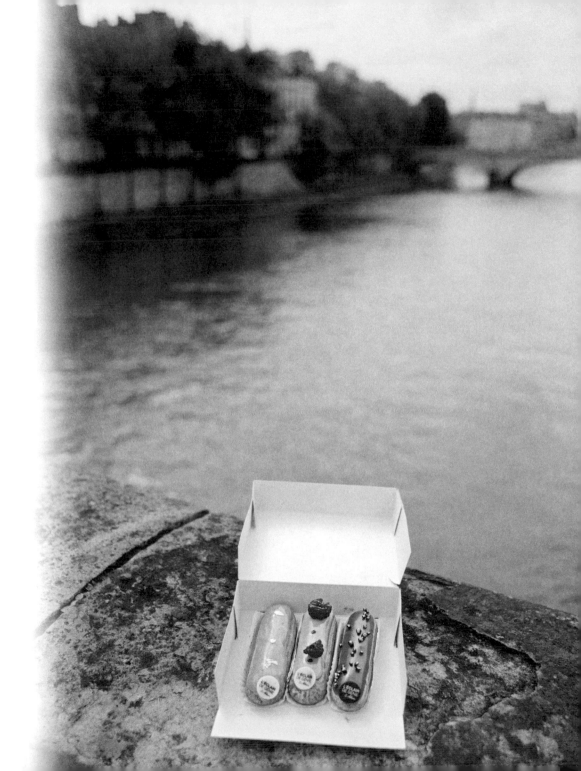

THE FRENCH ART OF TEA

While living next to Mariage Frères, I fell in love with drinking tea. There's just something luxurious about sipping a fragrant tea from a faraway land, even if you're lounging on your couch. I still make a pot of tea at least three to four times a week, and it's almost always a blend from Mariage Frères. It transports me to Paris even when I'm thousands of miles away. The French, starting with Mariage Frères in the Marais, turned drinking tea into an art form.

Mariage Frères was founded in 1854 by the Mariage family. One of the most historic and special places in the Lower Marais, this tea salon is the company's original location and France's oldest *salon de thé*. With its Colonial countertops, vintage scales, and old China tea chests, there is no better place in Paris to learn about and experience the French Art of Tea.

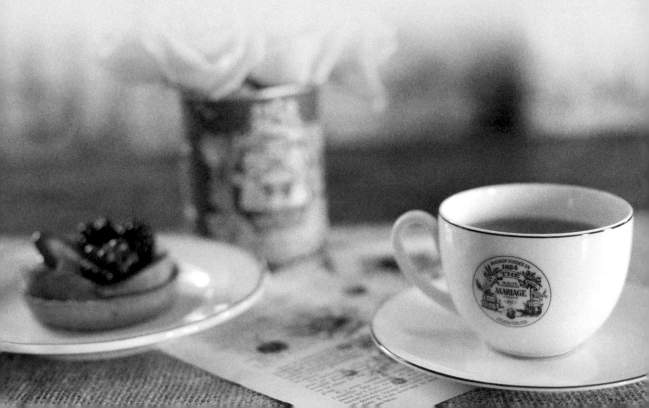

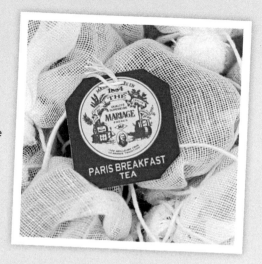

While the Japanese host spiritual tea ceremonies, and the British are known for their "afternoon tea," the French also have their own set of practices. This French ritual of tea drinking is based on the proper blending of teas, matching culinary delights to go along with them, and setting an elegant scene. The French pay attention to every detail. Water, teapot, and steeping time are all important steps in preparing the finest pot of tea. The type of teapot you select to serve your tea in is just as important to the foods served along with it. At Mariage Frères, you can buy these items and ask the tea sommelier to suggest which of their special blends pair well with each meal and type of dish, from seafood to spicy and desserts.

Many tea purists around the globe drink tea without adding any milk or sugar. However, according to the letters of Madame de Sévigné, it was a Frenchwoman, the Marquise de la Sablière, who first started the trend of adding milk to her tea. Leave it to a Frenchwoman to make even drinking tea more rich and decadent.

One of the most important beliefs of the French is that tea is meant to be enjoyed in tranquil settings. So when you're in the Lower Marais, take some time to sit and enjoy what will surely be the most perfectly prepared tea and most elegant presentation that you will ever experience. When at home, invite some girlfriends over and teach them the French Art of Tea. Dean & DeLuca carries a small assortment of Mariage Frères's top-selling teas. Some of my personal favorites are Lover's Leap, Marco Polo, Eros, Le Voyageur, Casablanca, and Wedding Imperial. When I'm not drinking a blend by Mariage Frères, it's always one from Tantalizing Tea, who not only creates wonderful teas but also sells my favorite selection of yixing teapots.

Hôtel de Ville

Paris's Town Hall Square is a great place to people watch and make new friends, including some single French men. Beach volleyball, ice-skating, and a live broadcast of the French Open are just a few of the seasonal activities the city hosts to bring Parisians together in this inspiring square.

Pain de Sucres
14, Rue Rambuteau

This decadent pastry shop offers some sweet confections and tasty savory treats. If the colorful homemade marshmallows in flavors like whiskey or matcha green tea don't grab your attention, biting into the flaky *pain de sucres* special filled with rosemary and tomato certainly will.

Le Défenseur du Temps
8, Rue Bernard de Clairvaux

Half a block past the Georges Pompidou museum you'll find this tiny passage. Look up to see a quirky brass and steel clock with a dragon, crab, bird, and soldier on the wall of the building. Notice the belly of the dragon moving in and out with his breath, counting the seconds of the day. Every hour from 9 a.m. until 10 p.m. the soldier is attacked by the crab, the dragon, or the bird, and a battle ensues. Such a magical neighborhood secret!

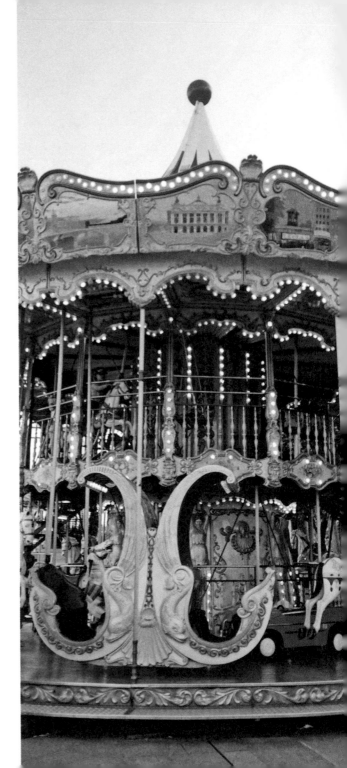

CENTRE POMPIDOU +
MUSEE NATIONAL D'ART MODERNE
Place Georges Pompidou

Not just for visiting inspiring works of art by Pollock and Dalí; the short-term exhibits are always a must-see. You'll also spot the neighborhood girls in the art house cinema, concert hall, and bookstore.

DINE AT GEORGES Located on the top floor with an exceptional view of the city. Dine next to Parisians who enjoy a delicious power lunch or like to show off hot dinner dates. You may recognize the signature clear fiberglass chairs from *Sex and the City* when Carrie Bradshaw met Aleksandr's ex-wife here for lunch. In *Le Divorce*, it was the location for the first of many decadent lunch rendezvous Kate Hudson shared with her "uncle-in-law."

LA FONTAINE STRAVINSKY Around the corner from the museum, you can snap photos in front of one of the fun moving sculptures, often a location for fashion editorial shoots.

Bazaar de l'Hôtel de Ville (BHV)
52, Rue de Rivoli

This department store is your resource for just about anything you could ever possibly need in Paris. Think of it as a Bloomingdale's, Target, Duane Reade, and Home Depot all in one. It's a great place to pick up all the best home décor items that you'll never find back home. I especially love roaming the aisles of the basement hardware department. I always pass a slew of Parisians picking up interesting items for their home—house keys, lightbulbs, furniture hardware, signs in French, and so many other items. For clothing and accessories, you'll find everything from Sandro to Topshop and be able to shop the collections without busloads of tourists being dropped off each afternoon. When you're all done shopping, head up to the rooftop bar, Le Perchoir du Marais.

Le Renard
12, Rue du Renard

The former art deco cabaret, Le Théâtre du Renard, is now a Marais girl's go-to spot for karaoke. Parisian girls sing karaoke, you ask? But of course, when it's the world's chicest karaoke bar. Enjoy delicious Asian food for dinner and chic cocktails, and sing along until 4 a.m.

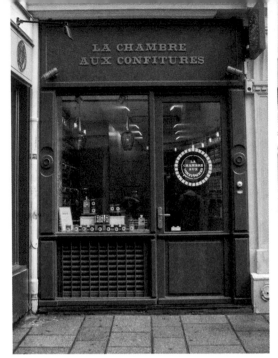
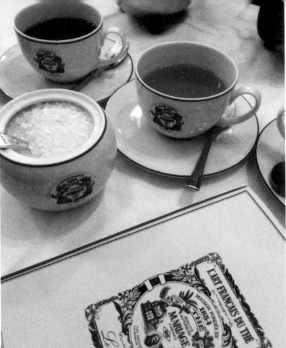

RUE DU BOURG TIBOURG

I was fortunate enough to live on this enchanting cobblestone street. It's without a doubt one of my favorite streets in Paris. Almost exclusively pedestrian, it remains quiet and a bit magical. With too many special places on one block to name, here are a few of my favorites, which I still frequent.

Le Coude Fou
No. 12

This is one of those "local" spots with some of the tastiest hearty French food I have ever put in my belly. A special treasure I have been enjoying for more than thirteen years.

Lizard Lounge
No. 18

Wander down the concrete steps to a lively cellar bar. Enjoy the cocktails or beer and have a chat with the English-speaking bartenders. All are from the U.S., U.K., or Australia and will recommend the cool new bars and hipster spots in Paris.

Mariage Frères
No. 30

As you open the door, you will instantly breathe in the aroma of more than five hundred selections of loose-leaf tea. Once seated in the dining room, you'll think you have arrived in colonial India. Let the gentlemen in ivory linen suits help guide your journey in selecting whatever type of tea you can imagine. Decadent tea-infused desserts add to the special experience when dining in France's first tea salon. Before you leave, pick up some fresh tea to bring home. Learn the French art of tea that all Marais girls are taught to know and apply to their daily routine.

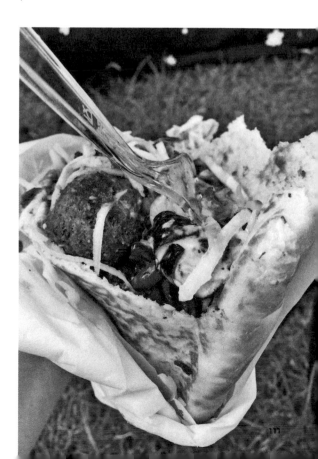

Tabio
15, Rue Vieille du Temple

My friend Christina (aka blogger TropRouge) has a deep obsession with socks, even in the summer months. She sent me here for the cutest stockings, tights, and socks in a variety of colors, styles, and fabrics. You'll find everything from bows to stripes, and a rainbow of colors in cashmere, lace, and wool. Have your initials embroidered on your favorite styles—it will take only a few minutes.

Johanna Braitbart
26, Rue des Blancs Manteaux

Play dress-up in Johanna Braitbart's delicate feathered headpieces and hats of all shapes and sizes. Chances are she will be in the boutique and will help you select the perfect piece to complement your style.

Suncoo
22, Rue des Rosiers

Sweet clothing and dainty accessories with a bit of an edge fill this boutique by the emerging Parisian brand. Let's keep this one a secret before it ends up all over the U.S.

Les Philosophes
28, Rue Vieille du Temple

When I'm craving a glass of wine, I love to get a table outside here and people watch. (Heat lamps are key in chilly months.) With your wine, a cheese and meat plate arrives.

L'As du Fallafel
34, Rue des Rosiers

Shopping works up an appetite, so hop in line (even when it's long, it moves quickly) for the most delicious falafel in all of Paris. Always top with their spicy sauce as it brings together the crispy falafal, eggplant, and the best hummus you'll ever taste. You can thank me later.

THE LOVE OF SANDRO

For years, when I have thought of chic Parisian style, the first contemporary collection that has come to mind is Sandro. It's chic, modern, and sexy, but never over the top. Designer Evelyne Chetrite stays true to the classics, updating timeless silhouettes with lace trim, cool cutouts, and interesting fabrics to create collections you can continue to wear for many seasons. Her accessories are equally chic and complement a look without overpowering it.

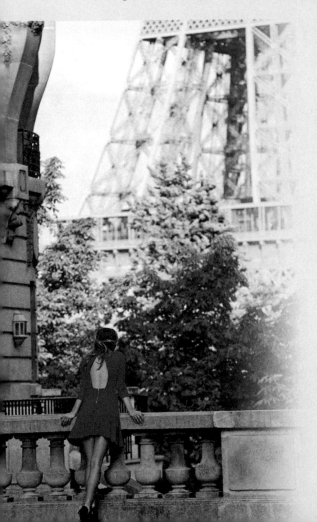

When I first thought of wardrobe for the *Bright Lights Paris* cover shoot, there was no doubt that it had to be a head-to-toe look from Sandro. But selecting a cover image was no easy task. No matter the style— from a red dress with cool cut-out back, a tea-length sheath dress with sheer panels, black and white pleated dress, or a sleek black jumpsuit with lace sleeves—Sandro's designs are all quintessentially chic and Parisian.

It's the type of collection where you can pair a sexy leather miniskirt with a delicate lace-trimmed blouse and create the perfect date-night look, or add a leather jacket to any dress and be set for the perfect fall dinner on the Seine. And can we discuss these boots? Even with such distinct and different pieces from the collection, from the ladylike to the sexy, they all look incredible with everything. Parisian women have rather small wardrobes, but they purchase versatile pieces to pair with many different looks. These sleek boots are a perfect example and made styling the cover so easy.

Although I'm sure all Parisian women have a few Sandro pieces in their closet, it's the Lower Marais girl who I believe identifies the most with the collections. One of my favorite Sandro locations to shop at is in the heart of her neighborhood, on rue Vieille du Temple.

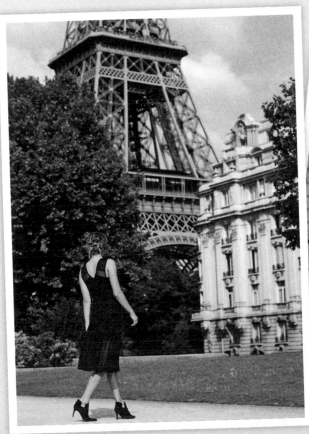

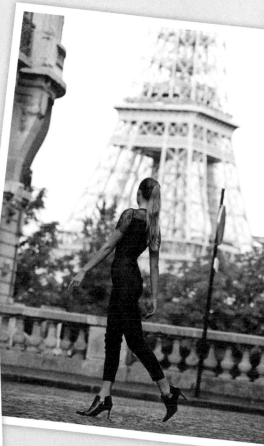

THE GOLDEN TRIANGLE OF THE MARAIS

This corner in the Marais is the place to find the Lower Marais girl's rock 'n' roll chic look for day and night. With five of my favorite boutiques in Paris for clothing and accessories that are more within my budget than luxury boutiques in Trocadéro, I like to think of it as *my* Golden Triangle.

Maje
49, Rue Vieille du Temple

Designer Judith Milgrom began designing Sandro collections with her sister, Evelyne, before branching out on her own to create Maje. Her collections are all rock 'n' roll glamour, a bit more daring but always chic.

Iro
53, Rue Vieille du Temple

Iro designers create laid-back, cool collections like no one else. They fuse edgy casual wear with classic stylish silhouettes and some of the coolest leather jackets in the best shades for both spring and fall.

Sandro
50, Rue Vieille du Temple

Chic and feminine with a hint of rock 'n' roll.

Barbara Bui
43, Rue des Francs-Bourgeois

Collection of ready-to-wear and accessories. Her elegant and modern styles infused with a bit of an edge makes women feel confident and sexy.

Bobbies
1, Rue des Blancs Manteaux

One of my favorite shoe collections for springtime loafers, summertime sandals, and fall booties, they offer great colors and fabrics and cute bow accents. And I love that it's still a Parisian girl's secret. Though I fear not for long.

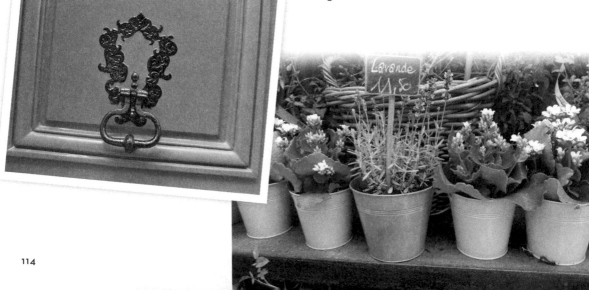

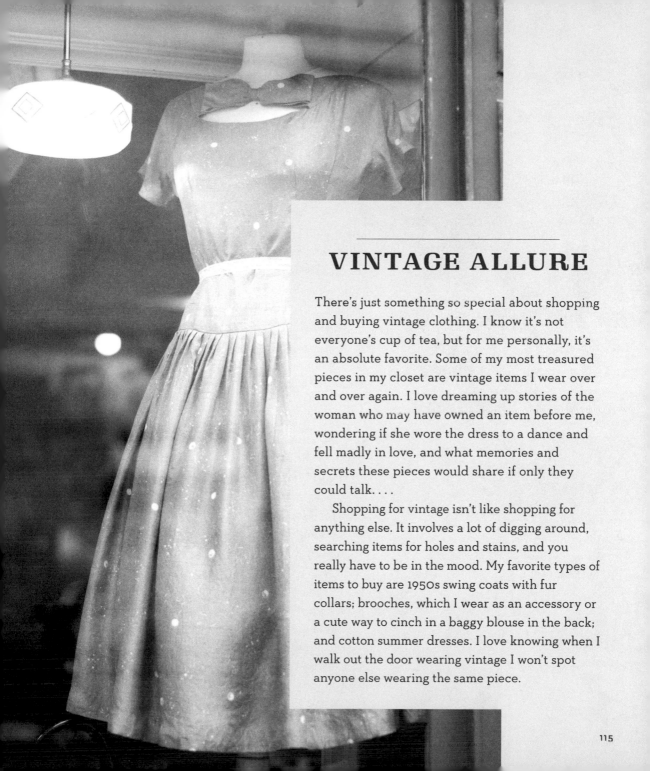

VINTAGE ALLURE

There's just something so special about shopping and buying vintage clothing. I know it's not everyone's cup of tea, but for me personally, it's an absolute favorite. Some of my most treasured pieces in my closet are vintage items I wear over and over again. I love dreaming up stories of the woman who may have owned an item before me, wondering if she wore the dress to a dance and fell madly in love, and what memories and secrets these pieces would share if only they could talk. . . .

Shopping for vintage isn't like shopping for anything else. It involves a lot of digging around, searching items for holes and stains, and you really have to be in the mood. My favorite types of items to buy are 1950s swing coats with fur collars; brooches, which I wear as an accessory or a cute way to cinch in a baggy blouse in the back; and cotton summer dresses. I love knowing when I walk out the door wearing vintage I won't spot anyone else wearing the same piece.

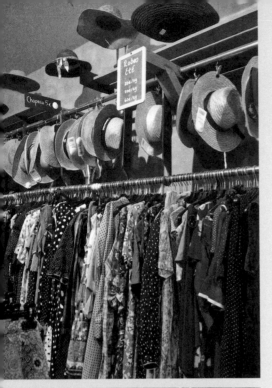

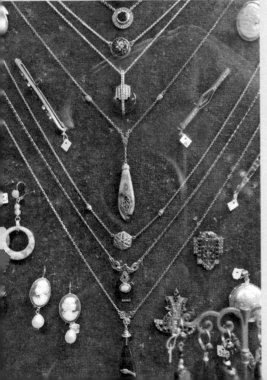

You can find unique vintage clothing and accessories online at eBay and Etsy. When buying vintage clothing online, pay attention to measurements and don't shop by size. A size 6 from the 1960s is far different from a size 6 today. Accessories are a safer bet when buying online since there are no sizing issues, aside from shoes. If you have a question about an item's condition, don't be afraid to ask the seller to send you additional photos besides what is being shown online. Sometimes you can score some gems at your local thrift store and yard sale, as well. The area of Florida where I grew up is a haven for Northerners when they retire. Areas like that are gold mines when shopping for impeccable vintage clothing and accessories, since the former Northerners no longer need their winter and more formal pieces in their Florida wardrobe.

Lower Marais women love to have a unique style all their own. To achieve that look, they regularly go vintage shopping for clothing and accessories. Lucky for them, they live in the best neighborhood for it, with a large assortment of boutiques selling vintage at all price points. Most are very affordable, with a few specializing in designer vintage items well worth the price.

Here's a curated list of vintage boutiques (shared by my Lower Marais girlfriends).

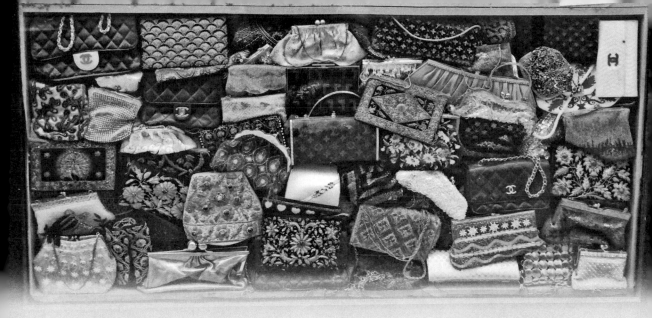

Mam'zelle Swing
35, Rue du Roi de Sicile

A sweet little vintage boutique in the Marais with a well-edited collection of clothing and accessories from the 1900s to the 1960s. It won't feel overwhelming like a lot of other boutiques that are packed full of merchandise.

Noir Kennedy
22, Rue du Roi de Sicile

A well-curated mix of rock 'n' roll vintage and new indie brands will have you pairing your skinny jeans with a vintage letterman cardigan. Don't freak out as you step into a coffin or an old British phone booth to use as a fitting room.

Coiffeur Vintage
32, Rue de Rosiers

Small but good. This is actually accessory heaven: they have countless cool belts and a good assortment of unique shoes.

Rag et Vertige
83–85, Rue Saint-Martin

One half of Rag focuses on more casual items like pilots' jackets and 1970s shirts and heels; the other side is more chic with vintage Hermés scarves, a 1960s Paco Rabanne dress, or a Gucci accessory.

SHOP BY WEIGHT

Take a stroll down rue de la Verrerie and you'll spot two fantastic shops where you can buy items in bulk and pay per kilo (pound).

Kilo Shop
69–71, Rue de la Verrerie

Everything is merchandised by style and trend.

Free'p'star
61, Rue de la Verrerie

This shop is a bit more of a mess, but is totally worth a rummage. In each area, you'll find baskets and scales to weigh your items so you know how much you're spending.

Vert d'Absinthe
11, Rue d'Ormesson

Absinthe boutique where you can shop and learn the history of this exotic liquor. A great spot to pick up gifts for the man in your life who loves making cocktails.

Carven
8, Rue Malher

Creative director Guillaume Henry designs the chicest of chic ready-to-wear and accessory collections. He's perfected a way to dress women in strong statement pieces, and no matter how strong the look, they still always look and feel feminine.

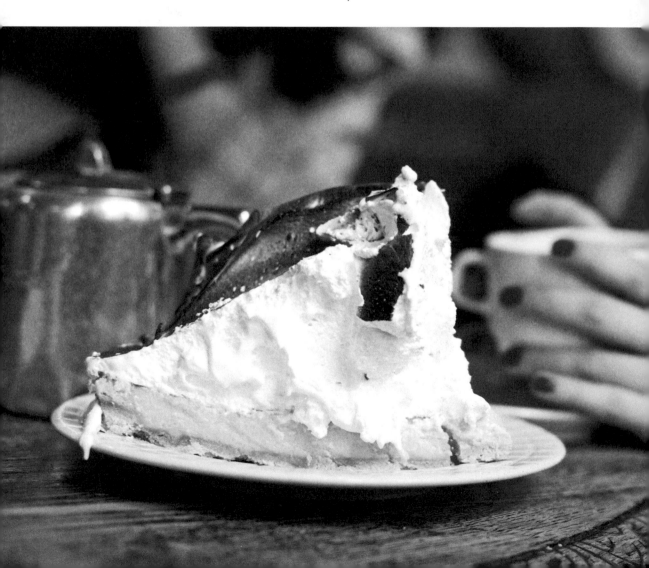

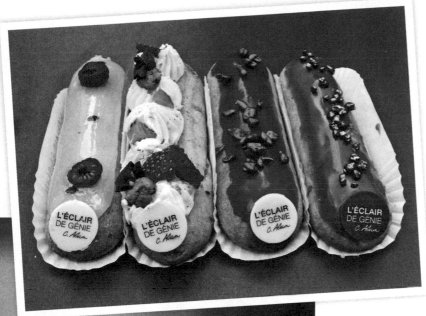

L'Éclair de Génie
14, Rue Pavée

Éclairs had never been my favorite dessert. I didn't dislike them; there were just many other types of dessert I loved more. That is until my first time biting into the éclairs at L'Éclair de Génie. They are absolutely, 10,000 percent worth all of the hype and Instagram selfies. Christophe Adam continues to add sensational desserts in exotic flavors to his menu, including ice cream éclairs and bonbons. I can't wait to taste what he comes up with next.

Au Petit Thai
10, Rue du Roi de Sicile

Get cozy in this adorable neighborhood restaurant with some of best Thai food in Paris. Just right for a girls' night or a romantic dinner with your beau.

La Loire dans la Théière
3, Rue des Rosiers

Since this is one of the most crowded Sunday brunch spots in the Marais, I like to arrive midmorning to beat the rush. Then we finish at the perfect time, when boutiques have just opened. I can't live without their French country food, flaky and savory tarts, and oh my goodness the homemade pies! You'll have such a tough time deciding which piece of pie to devour, so just order two different pieces!

PLACE DES VOSGES
NEIGHBORHOOD PICNIC SPOT

The oldest square in Paris is also the most magnificent. Take a break from a busy day to soak in the view of the arcade walkways and former homes of royalty. Daydream of Madame de Sévigné's life at no. 1 bis. Certain times of year, you'll come upon the sign "*Pelouse en Repos,*" meaning the lawn is resting and no one is allowed to picnic or lie on it.

MAISON DE VICTOR HUGO
no. 6

This opulent mansion of literary legend Victor Hugo shows his good taste in décor and breathtaking views of the park. Learn more about his stately life while he wrote *Les Misérables*, entertained friends like Alexandre Dumas, and spent time on the island of Guernsey, exiled for getting Napoléon III angry.

CARETTE
no. 25

A cozy tea salon with a scrumptious Mont Blanc pastry and a covered terrace overlooking the park. During the winter, warm up with a hot lemonade. In the mood for a quick lunch to eat in the park? Tasty salads and sandwiches can also be ordered to go.

—Mathilde Thomas, COFOUNDER OF CAUDALÍE PARIS

My favorite neighborhood to wander is Le Marais. Not only because there's a Caudalie boutique spa nearby but also for the ambience, all the little unique boutiques, and to eat at Carette café in Place des Vosges. Not far away, Le Musée de la Chasse et de la Nature is one of Paris's best-kept secrets.

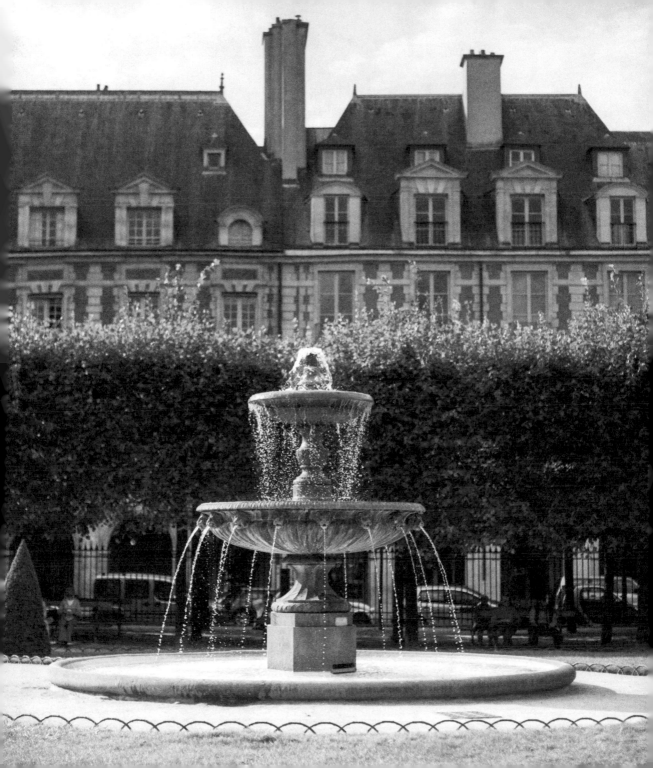

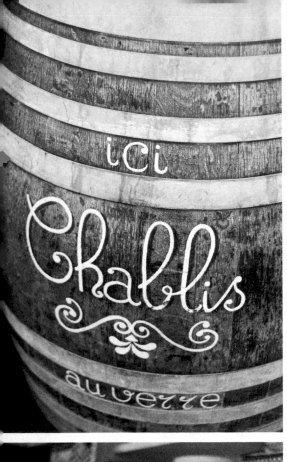

iCi

Chablis

au verre

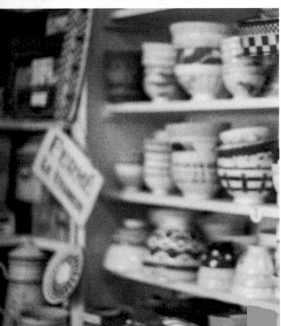

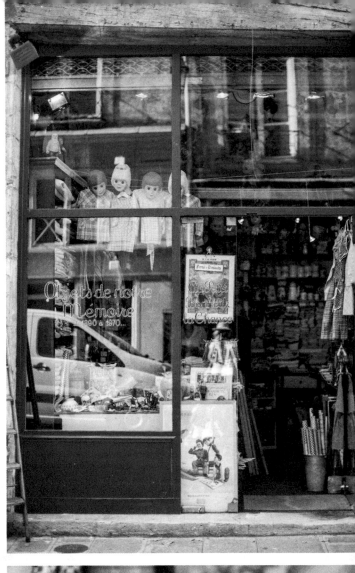

Objets de notre
Mémoire
de 1890 à 1970...

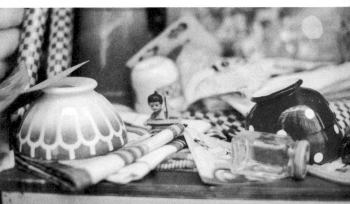

VILLAGE SAINT-PAUL

Take a walk south of the Marais between the river Seine and the rue de Rivoli and make your way to rue Saint-Paul. You will see what you think are ordinary passageways, but in fact they all lead you to the heart of this charming pedestrian-only village with antique, French artisan, and home décor boutiques. Shop for small items to bring home, get inspired to redecorate your pied-à-terre, and sit for a moment and enjoy the view.

AU PETIT BONHEUR LA CHANCE
13, Rue Saint-Paul
Stock your kitchen just like a Lower Marais woman with a mismatch of vintage kitchenware, colorful bowls, linens, and more. Full of vintage treasures for your home and entertaining, this store has a great collection of vintage holiday cards and parlor games.

LA PETITE MAISON DANS LA COUR
9, Rue Saint-Paul
This cute café, tucked away in the courtyard of the Saint Paul flea market, serves delicious homemade breads, quiche, and salads. If you are there in the winter, you must have their thick and creamy hot chocolate and let me know how you rate it against Angelina's.

CHEZ JULIEN
1, Rue du Pont Louis-Philippe
With a fantastic view overlooking the Seine and extra-tasty fries, this cozy bistro attracts all the cool Lower Marais girls.

PAPIER +
9, Rue du Pont Louis-Philippe
The French still have a strong appreciation and love for letting writing. Lower Marais girls stop by Papier + for handmade notebooks, paper, and note cards to carry on the tradition.

MAISON EUROPÉENNE DE LA PHOTOGRAPHIE
5-7, Rue de Fourcy
One of the most important photo museums in the world, where exhibitions change about every two months. Parisian girls get inspiration for their home, style, and life from the fifteen thousand contemporary photos from the 1950s to the present.

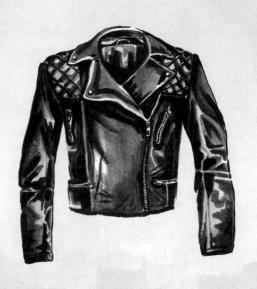

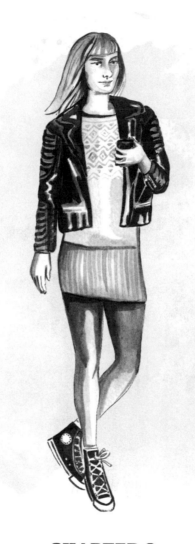

CHAPTER 6

UPPER MARAIS

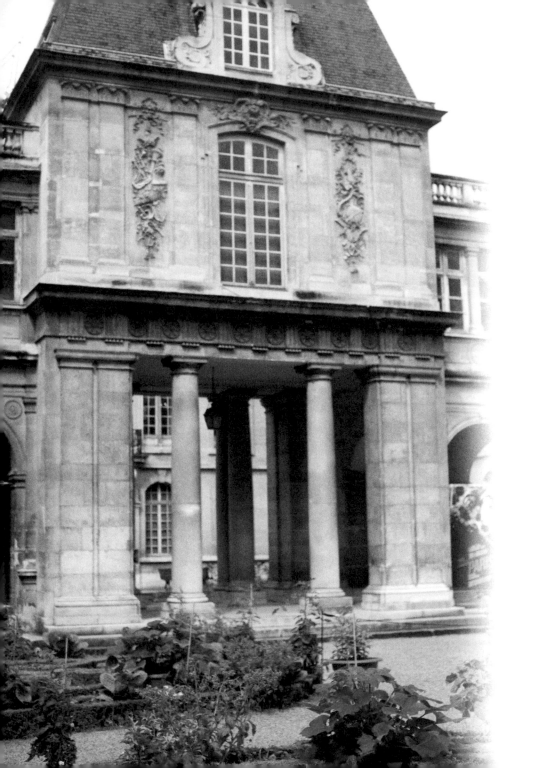

Like her arrondissement, the Haut (Upper) Marais girl is on the rise and in the know when it comes to style, food, and how to have fun. Located in the central bobo (hipster) hub, she's cool, chic, and a little bohemian—but of course not too much of either. Perhaps consider her the sister or cousin of the Lower Marais girl, with a little bit more edge. An art director working at a boutique agency, she takes more risk with her style but also remains very casual and cool. She's the girl who lives in her Converse but occasionally swaps them out for Chanel sneakers to wear with a black maxidress and leather jacket and, without question, pulls it off effortlessly. In this ensemble, she arrives fashionably late to the opening of the newest modern and contemporary art gallery on her block.

The Upper Marais girl is not afraid to move to a neighborhood when it's still up-and-coming and loves being the first of her friends to try the newest neo bistros and wine bars while still frequenting her longtime favorites, Derrière and Chez Omar. You can find her washing down oysters with killer cocktails at Le Mary Celeste, and when chocolate cravings kick in, she meets girlfriends at Chez Janou for the largest pot of chocolate mousse you'll find probably in all of France.

With some of the best specialty coffee shops and top baristas in Paris, her arrondissement can easily provide her caffeine fix at Fondation Café, Fragments, the Broken Arm, or the Boot Café. For a casual lunch with the guys, they meet up at Paris's oldest outdoor food market, Marché des Enfants Rouge, where they have their choice of authentic and inexpensive Japanese, Lebanese, Moroccan, or French fare and dine alfresco at the communal picnic tables.

She shops at quirky boutiques filled with artifacts and one-of-a-kind items. Merci concept boutique is her one-stop shop for all things cool, whether that's clothing and accessories for herself or her man of the moment, items for her apartment, or just to have lunch in their downstairs café. After, she may pop into Grazie, their hybrid pizza shop and cocktail bar, for an aperitif before heading home and getting ready for what's sure to be another late night on the town. She prefers to spend her time at underground cocktail bars, but don't dare ask her to mention any names—she likes to keep her hideouts a secret.

When friends come to town, she has them stay at Hotel de Petit Moulin, a charming boutique hotel designed by fashion designer extraordinaire Christian Lacroix. With a cute and mysterious boulangerie (bread shop) exterior, it's easy to miss. First on her list of neighborhood attractions are the Musée Picasso and the Musée Carnavalet, with a gorgeous garden courtyard and inside a tour of the history of Paris.

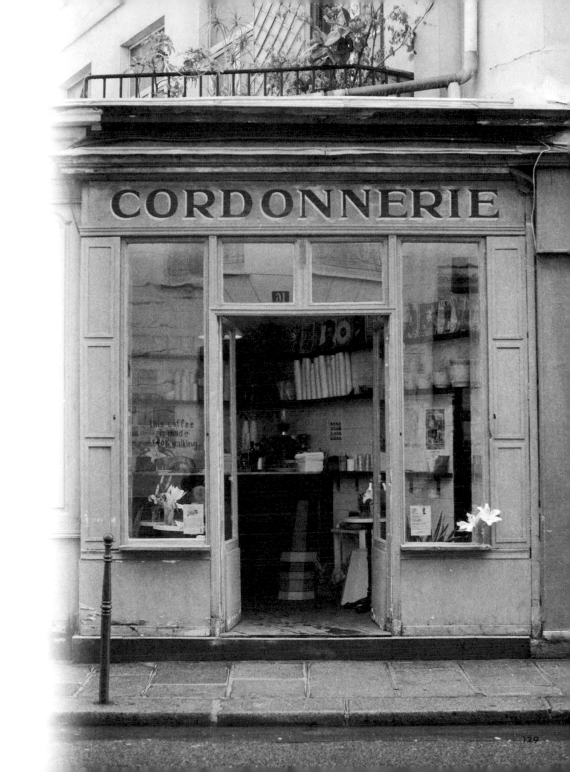

A NIGHT ON RUE DES GRAVILLIERS

A small, quiet block with a few of my favorite places all next to one another. Upper Marais girls have their choice of two great places for dinner, and a bar for drinks before or after.

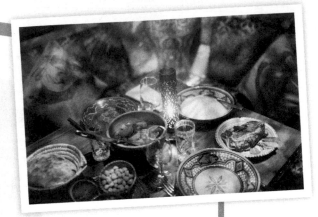

LE 404, no. 69
This Moroccan restaurant has incredible fig and lamb tagines and couscous. It's one I rarely skip and is fun with a group of friends and also dark and cozy enough for a sexy date night.

DERRIÉRE, no. 69
A beautiful town house turned restaurant. You could end up having dinner in a variety of rooms, like the bedroom or the living room. The food is delicious and is family-style eating, so best to enjoy with a group of friends. Play pool in the sitting room while you wait for your table to be ready in the dining room.

ANDY WAHLOO, no. 69
Moroccon kitsch bar. The Upper Marais crowd tends to arrive after 11 p.m., so make a Moroccan-inspired night of it and have dinner first at Le 404. After a few cocktails you may find yourself dancing on the banquettes.

Café la Fusée
168, Rue Saint-Martin

Overflowing with locals who all seem to know one another, this neighborhood café and bar is fun for lunch, dinner, or just to meet friends for a beer. I love their salads with fresh veggies and thinly sliced prosciutto, which I think pair perfectly with their fresh strawberry mojito.

The Broken Arm
12, Rue Perrée

Filled with the cool girls and guys of the Upper Marais, this concept shop boasts an organic café and coffee shop. Creatives stop in for the latest collaborations by Nike and Camper, exclusive Adieu loafers, and a curated selection of ready-to-wear styles by Raf Simons, Carven, Kenzo, Christophe Lemaire, and more.

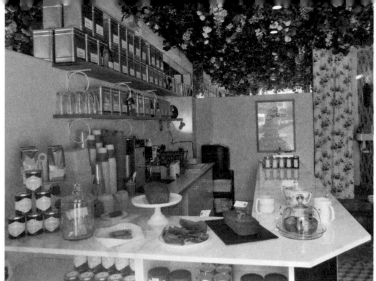
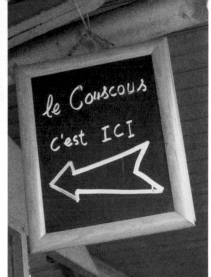

Lily of the Valley
12, Rue Dupetit Thouars

Parisian girls can't stay away from this lovely and tiny tea salon. As you enter Lily's secret garden, you'll be surrounded by flowers from the tapestry, wallpaper accents, and even flowers hanging from the ceiling. Enjoy her selection of fine teas and homemade breads.

Fondation Café
16, Rue Dupetit Thouars

Another fantastic addition to Paris's third-wave coffee culture. Upper Marais girls order their espresso alongside toast with fresh avocado.

L'Aller Retour
5, Rue Charles-François Dupuis

Keep your vegetarian friends away and surround yourself with locals at this hipster *bar à viande* (steak house). Retro interiors and great wine go well with the menu of incredible steak and roasted duck. Finish it off with a homemade strawberry tart.

Marché des Enfants Rouges
39, Rue de Bretagne

Hidden behind an iron gate is the oldest food market in Paris. In addition to fresh fruits and vegetables, there are stalls cooking everything from hearty French dishes to Moroccon couscous, fresh sushi, Italian pasta, and more.

Candelaria
52, Rue Saintonge

This tiny hot spot gets packed with Parisians who love Mexican street food. Once the homemade guacamole, tostadas, and tacos hit the spot, step behind an unmarked door at the back to find their speakeasy-style cocktail bar.

L'Îlot
4, Rue de la Corderie

With a well-priced menu composed almost entirely of chilled shellfish and seafood, you'll enjoy this gem located in a charming and quiet square in the Upper Marais.

—*Lauren Post*, BALLERINA WITH AMERICAN BALLET THEATRE

There are so many things that make Paris unique it is hard to pick just one! The lifestyle of outdoor cafés, reverence for good food, lots of red wine, coffee, and cigarettes are just a few things that make the city magical. I love the restaurant Chez Omar. They are known for their tagines with delicious slow-cooked meats nestled on top of delicate couscous. It is comfort food at its best. This is one of my favorite restaurants in Paris, especially in the winter or on a chilly, rainy day.

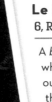

Le Barav
6, Rue Charles-François Dupuis

A *bar à vin* on a charming street corner, where you can actually reserve an outdoor table in advance. A favorite of the Upper Marais crowd, you can order wine at the bar or for a small fee go next door to their wine shop and pick up a bottle of your choice to bring back and drink.

Chez Omar
47, Rue de Bretange

A favorite of Upper Marais girls who stop in for lunch or dinner at this casual Moroccan restaurant. It's perfect for a group dinner with friends.

Al Taglio 2
27, Rue Saintonge

When the Upper Marais crowd craves fresh pizza, they stop into Al Taglio to pick up their favorite specialty flavors. All available by the slice or full pizza pie; my must have is "À la Truffle."

GET THE UPPER MARAIS LOOK

My favorite online boutique is Shopbop. Great jeans, new up-and-coming designers, and free return shipping! Read along to know how the Upper Marais girl shops and styles her look and you're sure to find it all on Shopbop.

Denim

The Upper Marais girl lives in her skinny jeans and wears them dressed up with heels or more casually with Converse sneakers. Pair them with just about anything: a solid black tee, a black-and-white striped sweater, or a silk floral printed blouse. J Brand, Current/Elliott, Rag & Bone, and Topshop are my favorite go-to denim brands.

Tees

I never use to think of T-shirts as a fashion staple until brands like Alexander Wang, Vince, and Current/Elliott started selling the best-fitting tees for all occasions that you can dress up and down with the right accessories. With the right pair of stilettos, skinny jeans, and a leather jacket you're set for a Friday night on the town. Graphic tees have also become a fun wardrobe staple, many with terms about Paris, or in the French language, that even Parisian girls approve of wearing. Check out SincerelyJules.com to find the latest styles from her collection.

Motocycle Jackets

This signature-style jacket is a staple not only in leather, but also in tweed, canvas, and knits. Depending on where you live, it can be worn almost year-round and will never go out of style.

Converse

You can really never have too many pairs of Converse sneakers—black, white, gray, and make sure at least one pair are high-tops. Unless you can afford Chanel or Isabel Marant sneakers, these are really the only kind, aside from a pair for the gym, that should ever be in your closet.

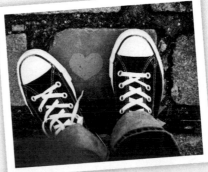

Hod
104, Rue Vieille du Temple

Accessory heaven for the Upper Marais girl, this multi-brand boutique sells jewelry and accessories from more than thirty designers and in a variety of prices.

Surface to Air
108, Rue Vieille du Temple

It's a concept store gone punk, and one of the best in the world. Even if it's not your style, pop in to see what's new in their selection of men's and women's collections. Chances are, the styles will trickle down and inspire even the most basic collections in seasons to come.

The Collection
33, Rue de Poitou

Specializes in cool wallpaper from British, French, and Scandinavian artists. Don't be afraid to pick up a roll for your home, as it should fit easily into your suitcase. Choose from trompe l'oeil, playful critters, screen-printed paper, and tiled mosaics prints. They also sell a quirky selection of home accessories, kitchen gadgets, and coat hooks.

Breizh Café
109, Rue Vieille du Temple

Whether she's in the mood for something sweet or savory, this is the Upper Marais girl's go-to for the best crepes in Paris. You're in for a treat with their homemade salted caramel sauce and melted Valrhona chocolate. Savory ingredients such as artisanal hams, herring roe, crème fraiche, and scallops create the perfect light and savory lunch.

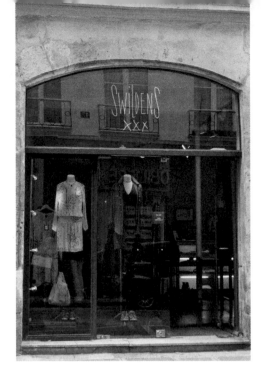

Swildens
22, Rue de Poitou

The Swildens collection encompasses all of the elements of an Upper Marais girl to help her create her perfect wardrobe. It's bohemian, romantic, chic, and rock 'n' roll all wrapped into one. The clothing is made of mostly natural fibers like silk, cotton, and wool.

Shine
15, Rue de Poitou

Multi-line boutique selling contemporary collections and their own in-house label. This was the first boutique in Paris to carry Marc by Marc Jacobs, and it continues that ideal by selling up-and-coming international designers mixed with staples from Edun, See by Chloé, and Cheap Monday.

Rose Bakery
30, Rue Debelleyme

Enjoy tea, fresh juices, and scones for breakfast or choose from the menu of organic assorted salads, quiches, and soup for lunch—all freshly made each day. When Parisian ladies want a break from cheese, baguettes, and pastries and instead need an extra dose of vitamins, they stop in for a fresh veggie platter.

Le Mary Celeste
1, Rue Commines

Look for Upper Marais girls to fill up this cocktail bar on any given night. Tasty small plates and oysters are paired with a stellar cocktail or Brooklyn Beer and the perfect way to start the night.

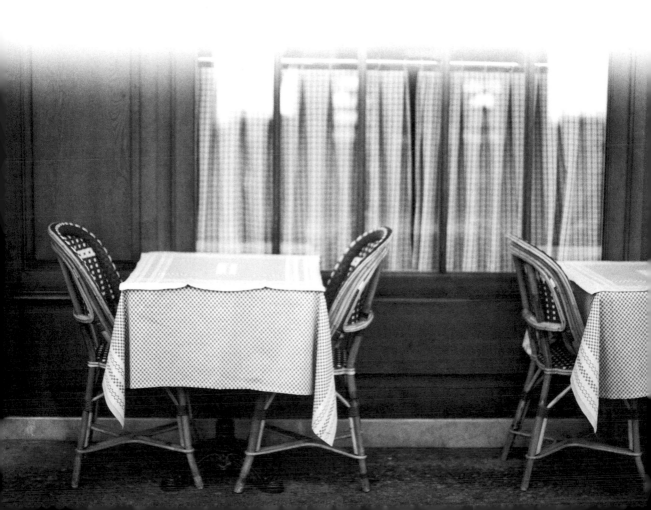

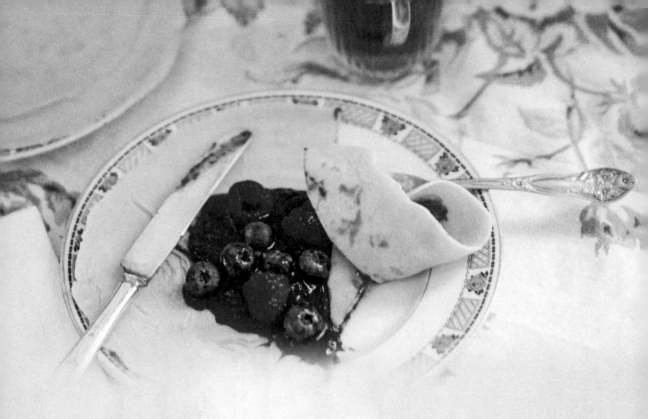

A SWEET PARISIAN ICON

I think the first dessert I ever associated with Paris was an ooey gooey Nutella crepe. Long before the obsession with macarons began, the first thing on anyone's mind when they arrived in Paris was biting into that first (of many) crepe. Watching the crepe man at the tiny stand on rue de Rivoli pour the batter and work his magic crepe wand to achieve a slightly crispy perfection, only to be followed by the smearing of heaping spoonfuls of Nutella hazelnut spread, was the best part of my day in Paris. Since that first trip many years ago, I have expanded my crepe eating to include savory, not just sweet, crepes. The Upper Marais girls have the absolute best location in Paris for crepes, Breizh Café. It's so good I recommend making a reservation if you're hoping to go for lunch or dinner.

On occasion I attempt to make my own at home. It took some practice, but once you learn the proper heat level you need for your skillet, crepes are quick and easy to make. When out-of-town friends are staying the weekend, I love to set up a table with different ingredients for a make-your-own-crepe breakfast.

Can't make it to the breizh? Make your own crepes at home:

French Crepes

- ¾ cup cold milk
- ¾ cup cold water
- 3 eggs
- 1 tablespoon granulated sugar
- 1 teaspoon vanilla extract
- 1 ⅓ cups all-purpose flour
- 5 tablespoons melted butter

In a blender, combine all the ingredients and blend for 1 minute on high. Refrigerate the batter for 2 hours.

Lightly brush a skillet with a tablespoon of vegetable oil or butter and place over medium-high heat. When the pan is just beginning to smoke, remove from heat, and pour ¼ cup of the batter in the middle of the pan. Quickly tilt in all directions for 2 or 3 seconds to evenly distribute the batter. Return the pan to the heat and, when slightly brown on the underside, flip the crepe over with a spatula onto the other side and cook for a few more seconds. Remove from pan and top with your choice of spreads (e.g., Nutella, peanut butter, Bonne Maman jams, etc.), sliced fruit, and a dollop of fresh whipped cream or a sprinkling of powdered sugar.

Ambali
79, Rue Vieille du Temple

The Upper Marais girl shops here for a unique piece to make her signature statement each season: a graphic-print belted swing coat with a tulip hem for winter or a versatile spring dress that with the right accessories can be girly for a work meeting or sultry on a Saturday night.

Robert et Louise
64, Rue Vieille du Temple

An old-fashioned tavern run by a father-and-daughter team. A giant fireplace where the meat is slowly cooked is next to a communal table. Bring your man, as he will love the meat-heavy menu and desserts made by Louise's grandmother. They offer one of Paris's best prix-fixe lunch specials.

Musée Carnavalet
16, Rue des Francs-Bourgeois

This sixteenth-century former hotel was the home of Madame de Sévigné and now houses a history of Paris museum, from the 1700s to present day. The collection includes personal artifacts, furniture, and paintings, and is a great stop for Marie Antoinette fans. The "Marie Antoinette Room" displays a lock of her hair preserved in a brooch, portraits painted just before her death, and even some of her children's favorite toys.

Gag & Lou Jewelry
38, Rue de Sévigné

Layer on their metal and embroidered bracelets. If you select a piece with a pendant, have them personalize it with your initials, which they can do on the spot.

Comptoir de L'image
44, Rue de Sévigné

This fashion photography bookshop was opened by a former assistant to Richard Avedon. Upper Marais girls browse through the archives and photography books for style inspiration.

Square Léopold-Achille
29, Rue de Sévigné

The center of the garden features pale peach-colored Île-de-France roses and a Maillol sculpture. Surrounded by a beautiful pink building covered in vines, it's one of my favorite squares in Paris. I like to bring a pastry or other sweet treat, take a seat on one of the benches, and imagine Madame de Sévigné walking through and gossiping with the ladies at court.

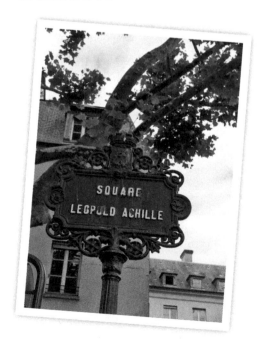

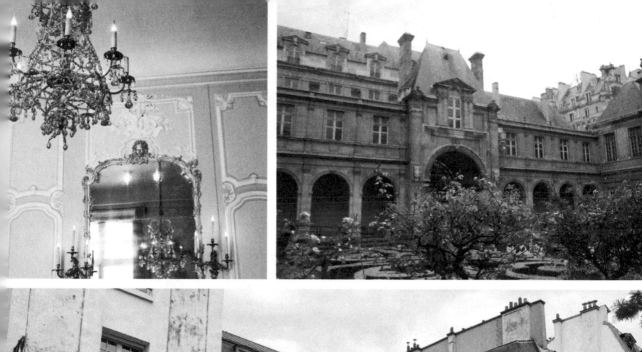

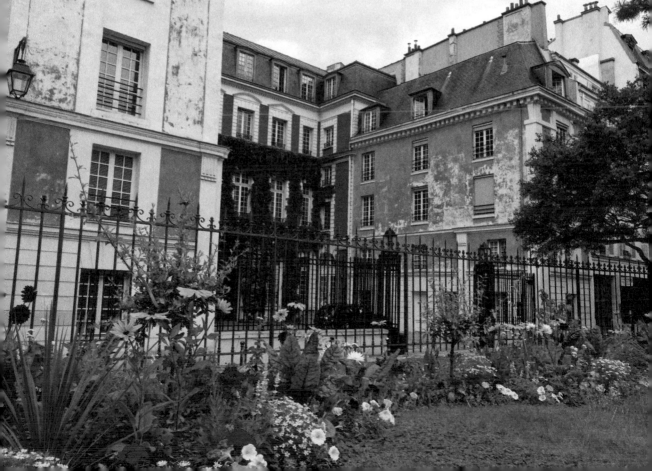

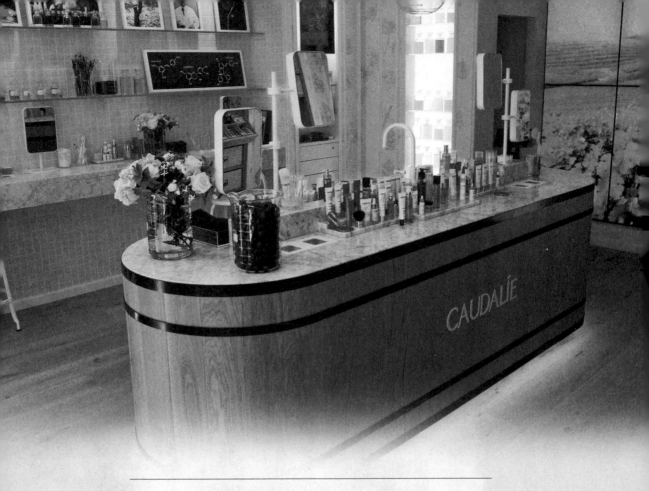

VINOTHERAPY

My drink of choice for just about any occasion is a glass of wine—whether
a buttery white Chardonnay, a red Châteauneuf-du-Pape, or a fresh rosé. It
tastes delicious, enhances the flavors or your meals, and even has a few
health benefits. When I heard that Caudalíe, the company who makes
many of my favorite French beauty products, uses nutrients in the grapes
and vines at their family vineyard in Bordeaux to make them, I had to learn
more.

By extracting powerful antioxidants from grape seeds, anti-aging
properties from vine stalks, and protective nutrients from wine yeast,

Caudalíe has developed patented products to protect, moisturize, and rejuvenate your skin. It's luxury from nature but at an affordable price.

Beauty Elixir is my first Caudalíe addiction, and for years I have had the regular- and travel-sized bottle in my bathroom. It's my favorite beauty item to use when I need to feel refreshed in the morning, before I go to bed, or when I'm on a long flight. It's definitely the Upper Marais girl's secret to getting the "just rolled out of bed but still look fabulous" glow.

A few of my other favorite products include the Divine Oil, Vinosource Moisture Cream, and Vinosource Serum, which I can't live without in the winter.

Their new collection of fresh fragrances is inspired by scents experienced throughout the day at their vineyard: Fleur de Vigne smells like morning dew; Zest de Vigne, high noon; and Thé des Vignes, an early evening breeze. Once you take in the scents of citrus fruit, fig, and jasmine, you'll want to book a flight to visit their vineyard, Château Smith Haut Lafitte, and Sources by Caudalíe Spa in Bordeaux.

For years I was jealous that French girls had such easy access to these products, but they are now available in the U.S., both online and at their flagship boutiques and spas in New York City and Los Angeles. I still love to visit their boutique in Paris, but it's fun to live near their taste of Bordeaux in the West Village.

Caudalie Paris, 8, rue des Francs-Bourgeois

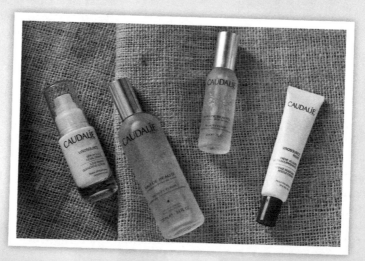

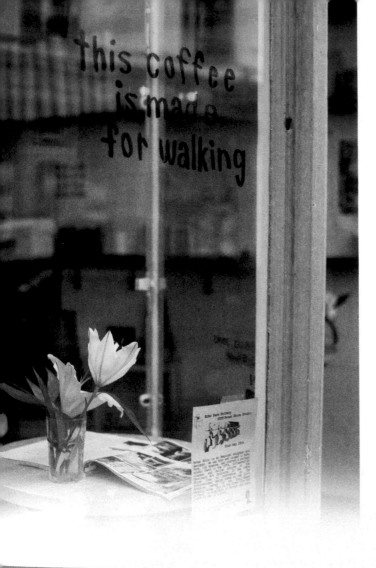

Chez Janou
2, Rue Roger Verlomme

A favorite of Upper Marais girls, it's one of their hideouts away from the tourists. You'll find Provençal French cooking with amazing ratatouille and something extra special about the chocolate mousse. I'll let it be a surprise.

Boot Café
19, Rue du Pont aux Choux

Located in the former shop of a *cordonnier* (shoe cobbler), this coffee shop may be tiny but the flavor isn't. Order yours to go like the locals and enjoy the rest of the day.

Musée Picasso
5, Rue de Thorigny

This beautiful museum houses one of the most complete collections of Pablo Picasso's works, put together in chronological order. It also includes his personal collection of paintings by Matisse, Renoir, and Cézanne, and a beautiful sculpture garden which you'll find Parisians roaming through on a sunny spring day.

—Fabrizio Moretti, DRUMMER OF THE STROKES

Every morning that I wake up in Paris, I'm overcome by the sheer contentment that beyond my doorstep bustles the greatest city in the world. I walk the streets looking upward like a lover spellbound, led by the famous beige rooftops that pierce the crystalline French sky, until I'm finally reminded, as if by a mental tap, that I'm headed to get coffee at my favorite Boot Café to start my day, and that this is not just my imagination.

L'Apparement Café
18, Rue des Coutures Saint-Gervais

Across from the Picasso Museum, this fantastic wine bar has a fun selection of board games. On a rainy night, join the Upper Marais girls, order a bottle of wine, and play a few rounds of Uno.

Clown Bar
114, Rue Amelot

Former cold-weather circus from the Belle Epoque era is now a delicious bistro and bar. They've kept the circus décor and added creative dishes with an all-natural wine list. Fried *bulot* snails are super-tasty—a favorite of Parisians to-go on a Sunday night.

Merci
111, Boulevard Beaumarchais

My personal favorite for best concept shop in Paris, and even any city that I've traveled to. Located in a former wallpaper warehouse, it's the coolest mini department store imaginable. From the clothing and accessories to furniture and kitchen gadgets, I want it *all*. Have tea in the Used Book Café, lunch at the downstairs café. Basically stay all day and see what the Upper Marais girls are buying.

Grazie
91, Boulevard Beaumarchais

All-in-one pizza and cocktail shop from the owners of Merci and just a few doors away. Their mad-scientist mixologist has created an extensive cocktail list that complements wood-oven pizzas prepared by some primo Italianos who know their pizza.

La Pharmacie
21, Rue Jean-Pierre Timbaud

The bright turquoise façade welcomes you to this delicious neighborhood neo-bistro. Because it was a former pharmacy, you'll spot antique pharmaceutical "curiosities" on display with bottles of wine. With a simple menu including only five options of appetizers, entrées, and desserts, you'll spend more time enjoying your friends than deciding what to order.

Au Passage
1, Bis Passage Saint-Sébastien

Even after the departure of chefs James Henry and Shaun Kelly, Au Passage is still a favorite of the neighborhood crowd. It's a super-relaxed atmosphere with delectable small plates that are fun for sharing. It should be illegal to not order the burrata with coriander flowers.

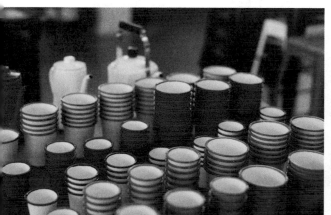
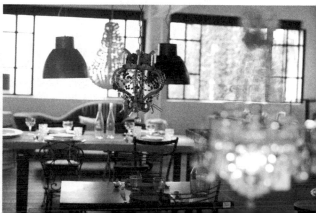

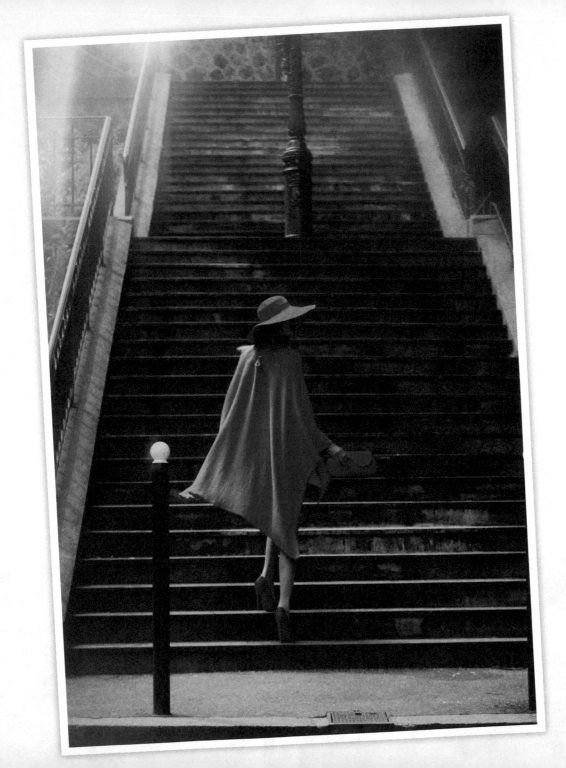

Guy Aroch

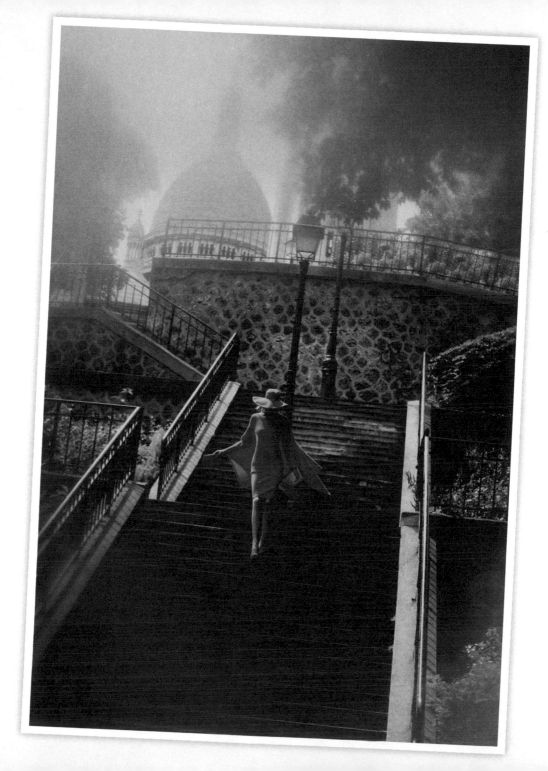

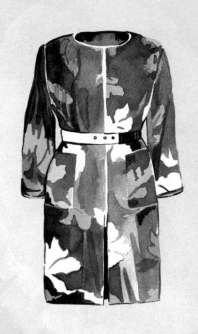

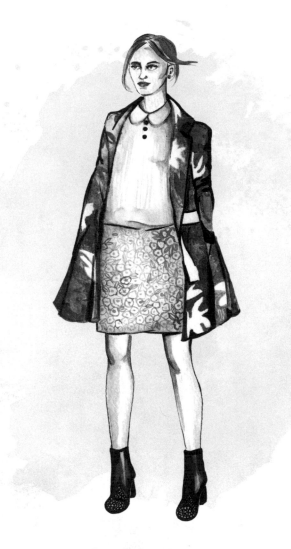

CHAPTER 7

MONTMARTRE

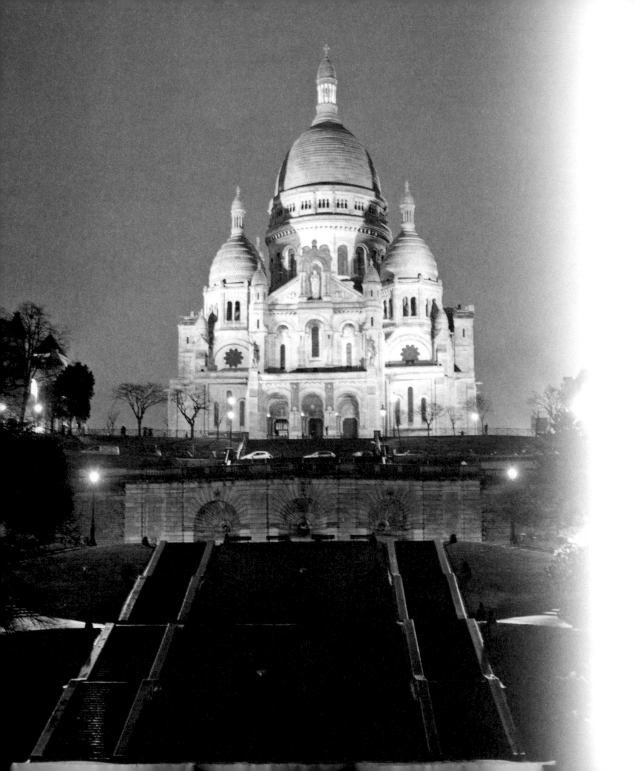

Paris is the most magical city in the world for so many reasons, one being the hillside village of Montmartre. Twisting cobblestone streets, romantic staircases, ivy-covered mansions, and picturesque rooftop views of the city are the perfect backdrop for the enchanting Montmartre woman. Her style is sophisticated and eclectic, in architectural silhouettes, artistic prints, and some menswear mixed in. Because she's not afraid to mix textures and prints both in her wardrobe and her home décor, you can always count on the Montmartre woman to have a unique look all her own.

Inspired by her neighborhood, which Renoir, Dalí, and some other artistic legends once called home, she may work as a curator at an art gallery in Saint-Germain-des-Prés. On her way home she saunters down rue des Abbesses in an Etro maxidress to meet friends at La Mascotte for oysters and rosé wine.

On weekends, she doesn't need to travel far, as there is a lot to do and see in her village. The hilltop is home to Paris's oldest vineyard, lovely windmills, and beautiful sunsets. In the fall, she joins the rest of her neighborhood friends at the annual harvest festival with a week of parades, dancing, and fireworks.

At the start of spring, the Montmartre woman spends a Sunday afternoon getting re-inspired in Giverny, strolling through Monet's gardens and around his water lily ponds. Seeing the wisteria-covered archways before the summer tourists arrive is a quiet retreat after a dreary winter.

Montmartre's winding cobblestone streets are where I imagine the French created *le flaneur*, which is to stroll and saunter aimlessly and without a destination in mind. It's the most perfect area to get lost in, along the back streets behind the Sacré Cœur, and let the spirit of the Belle Epoque guide your way.

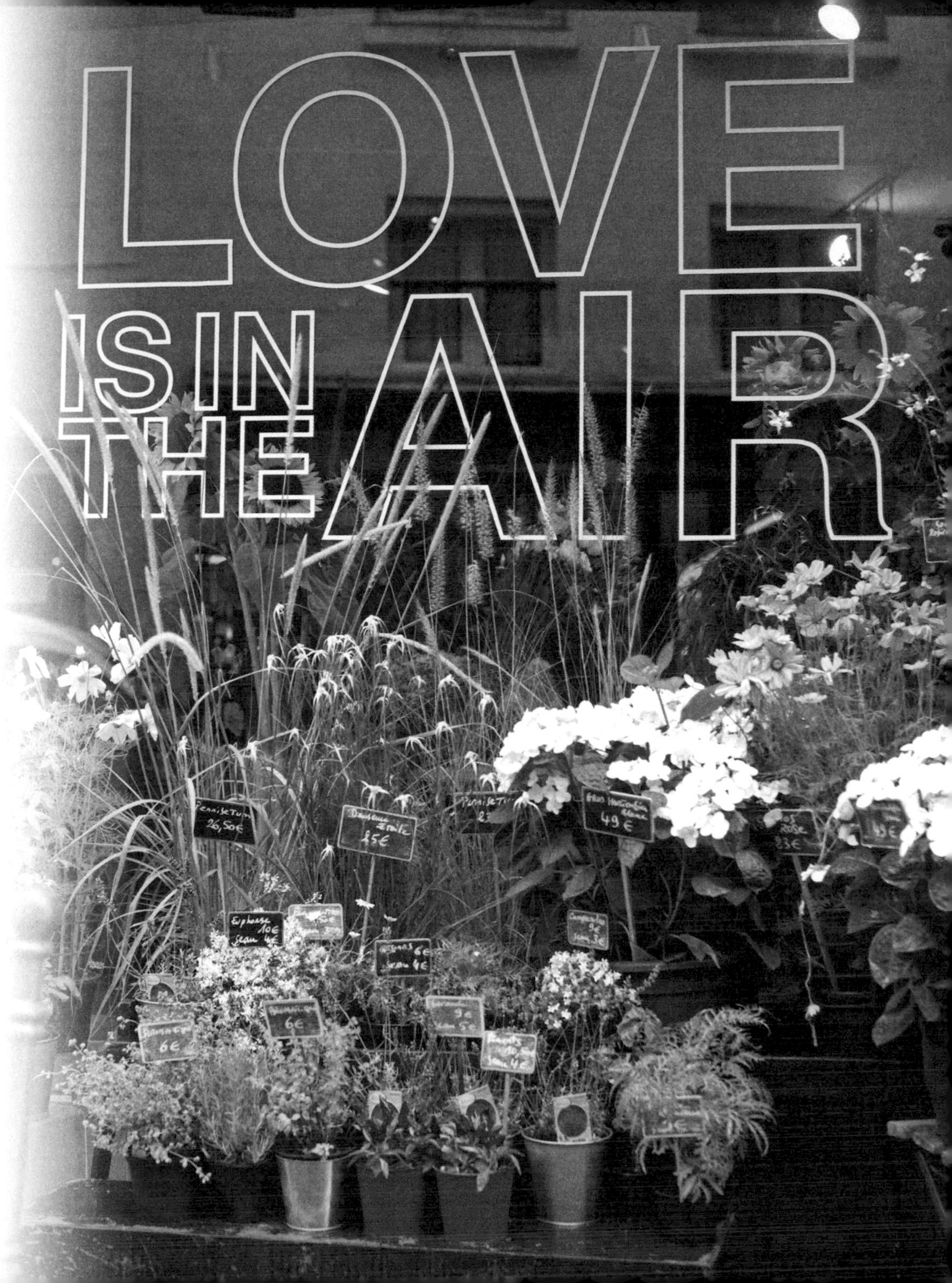
LOVE
IS IN
THE
AIR

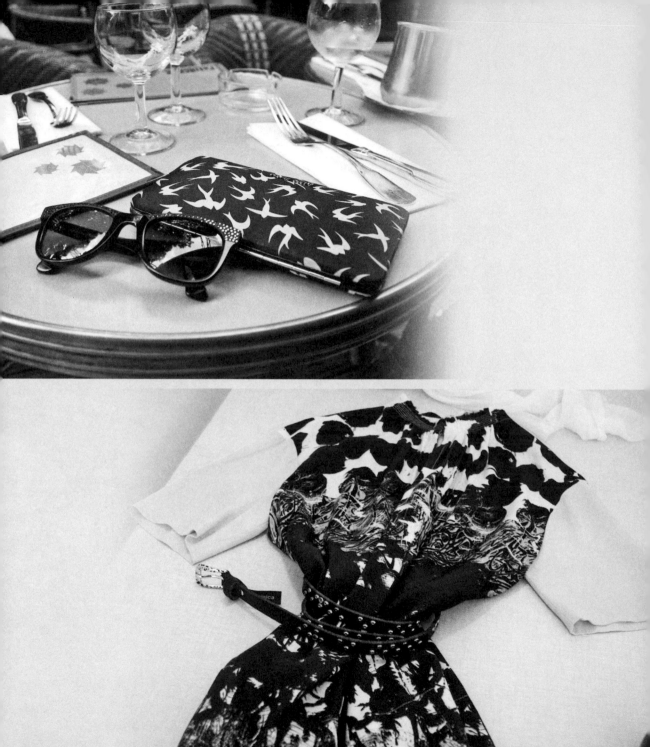

GET THE MONTMARTRE LOOK

Prints and Textures

Montmartre women aren't afraid of mixing prints or textures, and neither should you be. Try mixing silk florals with geometric or striped prints, or throw a wool plaid coat over a pleated chiffon maxidress.

Statement Coat

When I think of amazing statement coats, the first collections that come to mind are Marni and Prada. Each season, they design the most interesting coats, structured and architectural, in a wide range of fabrics, prints, and colors. You can definitely find more budget-friendly brands, but always look at these two collections for inspiration.

Oversized Clutch

The envelope clutch is not just a hot trend, but is here to stay. Accent an eclectic look with a solid-color clutch in a textured fabric, leather, or fur, or mix in a clutch in a complementary geometric or floral print.

Artistic Jewelry

Whether a cuff bracelet, earrings, or a necklace, distinctive jewelry is a must-have accessory for the artistic woman. Shopbop has the best selection of Gorjana and Adia Kibur pieces, with a large assortment that you can mix and match with daytime or nighttime looks. Splurge on a Dannijo necklace or cuff. Whether you wear it with a scoop-neck cashmere sweater or a cocktail dress, you're sure to turn every head when you walk into a room.

Chine Machine
100, Rue des Martyrs

This vintage boutique is where Montmartre ladies go to buy, sell, or trade their vintage pieces. They also pick up vinyl records and cool objects to decorate their home, like small vintage vases or lamps.

Mira Belle
6, Place Charles Dullin

Women of Montmartre have a special boutique where they can pick up beautifully designed hats for any occasion. Whether a simple and elegant cloche hat to wear every day, a 1920s party piece, an avant-garde creation to wear to the yearly Prix de Diane horse race in Chantilly, or something a bit more flamboyant and spicy, Mira Belle has the perfect chapeau.

Loft by Design
20, Rue Yvonne le Tac

Loft by Design offers simple architectural silhouettes in fine natural fibers. Maxi wrap skirts, cashmere cardigans, and wool tailored trousers are all a part of a Montmartre girl's daily wardrobe. When shopping for herself, she often picks up a sweater or button-down shirt for her beau.

Restaurant Miroir
94, Rue des Martyrs

A rustic neighborhood bistro full of charm, locals, and comfort food. No need to wait outside for a table; instead go across the street to their wine bar while you wait for one to be ready.

Ekyog
89, Rue des Martyrs

Not just a wonderful collection, Ekyog is also wonderful for the world, producing each piece using methods of sustainable fashion. From the sourcing to the fabrics and the sewing of the pieces, the collection of beautifully detailed artistic prints and easy-to-wear silhouettes is made using the finest organic cottons, soft renewable wools, linens, and more.

Belle de Jour
7, Rue Tardieu

Step into this beautiful art nouveau boutique where they sell and restore vintage perfume bottles, powder boxes, and other scent-related accessories. When you return home, you can spritz your perfume like the ladies of la Belle Epoque, when perfume was the ultimate symbol of luxury.

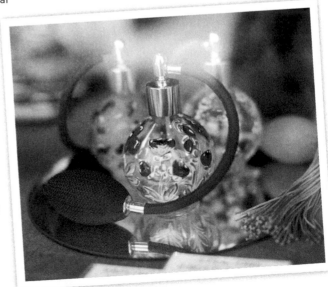

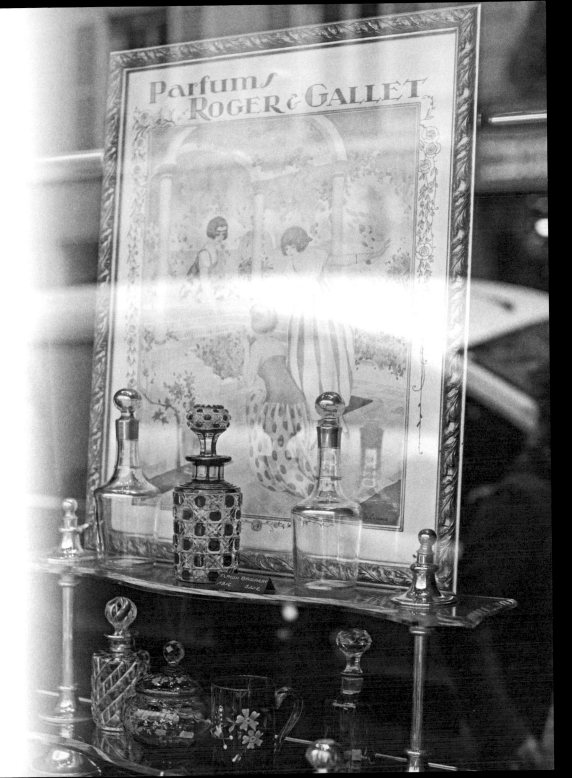

ART MEETS HOME DÉCOR

One of my favorite home décor stores in Paris, La Case de Cousin Paul, brings out a bit of my creative side, which is sometimes tough to do. My brain works in overdrive with marketing and strategy, but artistically . . . well, I've always needed a bit of help to pull that out of me. My friend Keiko Lynn, however, is super creative, and I always look at her blog and Instagram posts for style, makeup, and home inspiration. Lucky for me, when I first found La Case de Cousin Paul, it was while on a trip with Keiko.

The boutique is literally a shop full of home décor polyester balls in countless colors—beautiful bright, neutral, and jewel tones—which you then hook onto a strand of indoor lights. Homemade and lightweight, these lit balls are displayed in clear cylinder bins throughout the store.

You pick the colors you like and the length of the light strand, and then begin creating your personalized piece of home décor. Knowing the colors of my bedroom, Keiko helped me decide on a combination of turquoise, teal, silver, and light gray balls, while she put together the perfect combination of peach, mint, gold, and tan to complement the décor in her studio space, Brooklyn Brigade, which she shares with our friend Helena. I can't wait to return and select a new strand for my bathroom. The shop ships worldwide and offers light strands with your choice of European or American plugs.

The Montmartre woman's approach to home décor is similar to her personal style: mixing prints, textures, and different shapes to create a unique look. In her home, you'll find illustrations and paintings, sculptures, and different ways of lighting each room. She shops at flea markets, antique shops, and even buys new items to mix in with the unique pieces of the past. Her eclectic taste is always surprising but is never overpowering in her home.

La Case de Cousin Paul, 4, Rue Tardieu

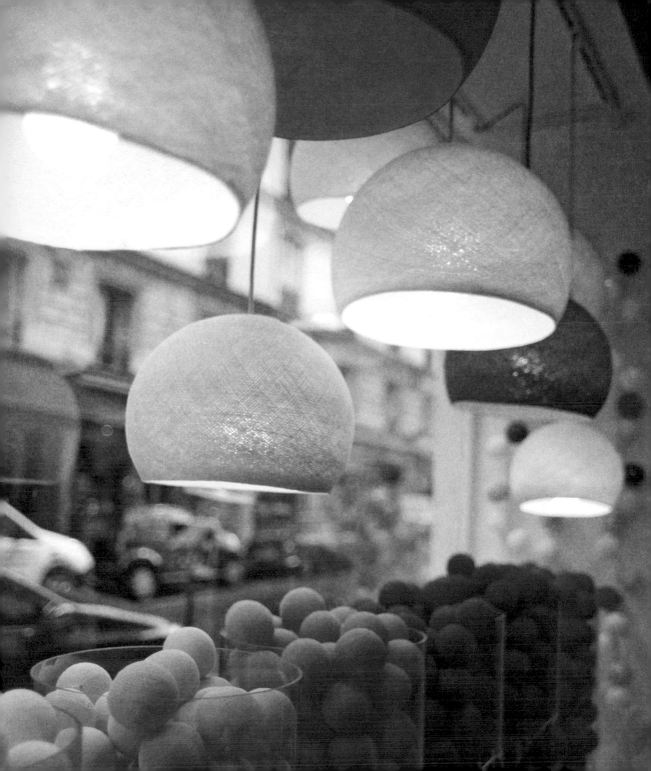

Spree
16, Rue la Vieuville

If there is one boutique in the area that to me perfectly captures the style and spirit of the Montmartre woman from head to toe, it's Spree. A mix of art gallery, exhibition space, and designer boutique, the curated assortment of both fashion and design furniture is always on point with what's happening in art and fashion. Pieces from Helmut Lang, Antwerp designer Christian Wijnants, and illustrator-turned–fashion designer Pierre-Louis Mascia help develop the Montmartre girl's look.

Jérémie Barthod
7, Rue des Trois Frères

Montmartre women appreciate art they can wear as much as the objets d'art that adorn their home. Barthod's wrist cuffs, earrings, and necklaces are so unique that you just need one piece to turn any outfit into an ensemble worth noticing.

Le Refuges des Fondues
17, Rue des Trois Frères

This legendary fondue restaurant with a quirky twist was made famous in part by the movie *Amélie*. The Montmartre woman doesn't go often; she saves it for occasions when friends are visiting from out of town and in the mood for a fun and novel experience. Be prepared for a lively do-it-yourself meal while drinking wine out of a baby bottle.

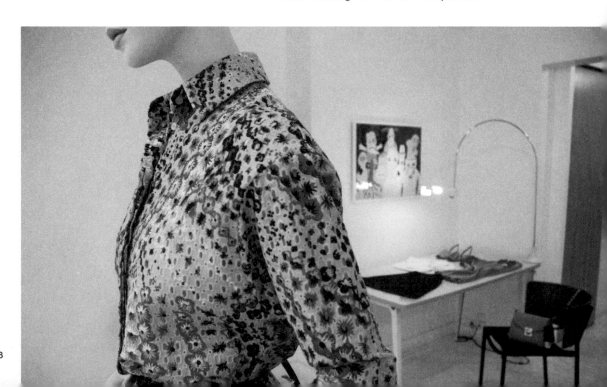

La Famille
41, Rue des Trois Frères

When they've finished shopping for new, artistic pieces for their wardrobes, Montmartre girls head here for artistic cocktails. The bar is famous for their Molecular Mojitos in different fruit flavors, which are served with their own edible accessories. While these cocktails are delicious, the best part may be when they first arrive smoking (with the help of dry ice) and topped with gummy eyeballs, chocolate pop rocks, or sometimes a syringe full of peach liqueur.

Etablissements Lion
7, Rue des Abbesses

Visit this gourmet shop to pick up all the ingredients you need to make delicious risotto, couscous, or tabbouleh. The prepackaged mixes contain quality spices and grains in one bag for easy preparation. And the cute packaging makes this a great take-home gift for friends who like to cook.

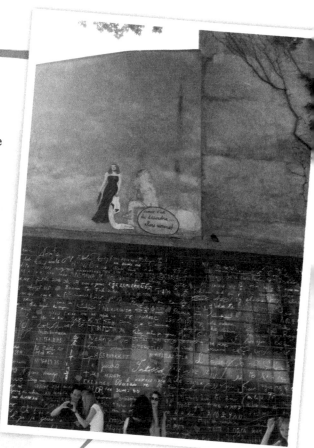

PLACE DES ABBESSES

Three must-see pieces of Montmartre history in one small triangular courtyard.

EGLISE SAINT-JEAN-DE-MONTMARTRE

Beautiful church with gothic vaulted ceilings and an art nouveau stained glass mural.

ABBESSES METRO ENTRANCE

One of only two Belle Epoque entrances designed by Guimard that are still left standing in Paris.

LE MUR DES JE T'AIME (I Love You: the Wall)

A mural of tiles by artist Daniel Boulogne with "I Love You" written in 250 languages. Go with your love and snap a selfie kissing in front of your favorite language of love.

Coquelicot
24, Rue des Abbesses

This boulangerie and café is decorated in bright red poppies—the blooms found wild in wheat fields. It feels like walking into your grandmother's home, except you can pick up baguettes baked fresh each morning by their three bakers. Make sure to sample the hot cocoa, specially made with rich pastry chocolate.

Chez Camille
8, Rue Ravignan

A bohemian café and dive bar with locals pouring out onto the street late at night, this is where Montmartre girls meet up on a Sunday afternoon, and sometimes stay for a game of Scrabble.

Beauty Monop'
28, Rue des Abbesses

This mini Monoprix (similar to our Target stores) exclusively sells beauty items, from nail polish and lipsticks to shampoo and conditioner, to skin care products. It's a quick and easy stop for the Montmartre girl to pick up refills of her daily beauty products.

La Cave des Abbesses
43, Rue des Abbesses

Here you can shop in the front and party in the back! Step through the door at the back of the wine shop to join the neighborhood crew for a glass of full-bodied red Burgundy, Corsican coppa, and assortment of fromage at this divey wine bar.

Guilo Guilo
8, Rue Garreau

One of the best Japanese restaurants in the city, it only serves dinner, and there is only one seating per night; making reservations a must. The small courses are brought out looking more like artistic gifts and less like your dinner. Reserve a seat at the counter so you can watch the chefs work their magic.

Café Burq
6, Rue Burq

This cool hipster bistro with simple décor serves food late into the night. The women of Montmartre always start their meal sharing the roasted Camembert with honey, and you should too.

Cinema Studio 28
10, Rue Tholozé

Montmartre's vintage cinema, where Cocteau films premiered in the 1940s, now shows current and vintage films. Ladies of Montmartre go early to have tea in the secret terrace café.

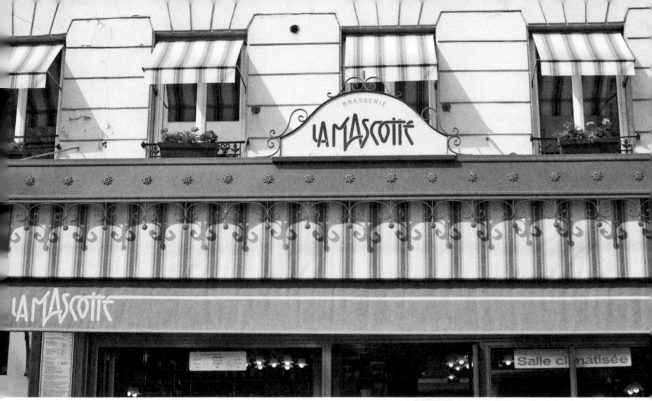

La Mascotte
52, Rue des Abbesses

The neighborhood men sit at the bar with their aperitifs listening to traditional French accordion tunes while the ladies sit on the terrace with a glass of rosé wine, both groups enjoying a platter of fresh oysters. One of Montmartre's most famous women, Edith Piaf, lived upstairs in this former Hotel Particulier.

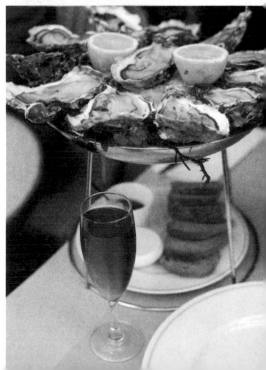

Les Petits Mitrons
26, Rue Lepic

Fresh berries, apples, or peaches on a crunchy crust make these some of the tastiest fruit tarts in all of Paris. You can pick up an assortment of mini tarts in different flavors.

Tombées du Camion
17, Rue Joseph de Maistre

If you're a collector of tiny unusual objects, then you'll love this quirky shop which sells multiples of vintage kitsch items like mini toys, dolls, glass eyeballs, and more that will remind you of your childhood. Pick up enough of one item to use as table settings for a dinner party.

Le Bal Café
6, Impasse de la Défense

Down a hidden alley in the Le Bal Exhibition Center and photography hall, this gem serves modern British fare. It's a neighborhood favorite for weekend brunch, with freshly baked scones, Welsh rarebit, and the tastiest sticky toffee pudding in Paris.

Gontran Cherrier
22, Rue Caulaincourt

Single ladies in Montmartre go to Gontran Cherrier's boulangerie for their weekly baguettes and pastries. Not just because he bakes interesting flavors (squid ink baguettes, anyone?) or because his baguettes are voted some of the best in Paris, but for a much more important reason: to catch a glimpse of and catch the eye of one of the world's sexiest bakers.

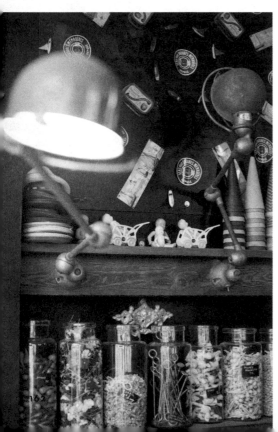

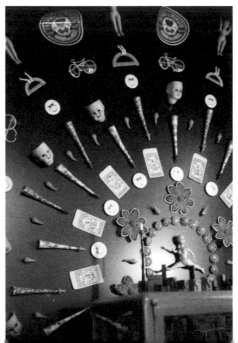

Jeanne B
61, Rue Lepic

When Montmartre women want to have dinner at home but don't feel like cooking, they stop by this epicerie, where you can eat in or take out freshly made meats and side dishes. Perched on a quiet section of rue Lepic, the tables outside provide a view of the village's windmill. The house specialty is their roast chicken, which they make each morning in the rotisserie oven.

Le Coq Rico
98, Rue Lepic

I pretty much love all kinds of food, but without fail my go-to favorite is usually the chicken dish. So when I heard about Le Coq Rico serving up almost nothing else but chicken, I had to have a taste for myself. Sure enough, some of the tastiest chicken, not just in Paris but across the globe.

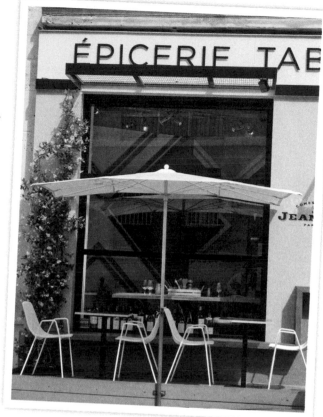

—Meghan Markle, ACTRESS AND FOUNDER OF THETIG.COM

I love that Paris always surprises me. No matter how well I think I know the city, I will spend a lifetime discovering something new about it. I love that. Le Coq Rico, tucked at the top of the hill close to Sacré-Cœur, is a gem serving up roasted chicken and frites. Yes, there are a few other options, but most come here for the blue-footed chicken (Poulet Bresse) which is as rare as it is delicious—it's worth the trek. Share a bottle of wine, snuggle into a booth, and have a perfect and simple meal of roasted chicken, frites, and salad. I'm serious when I say it's one of my favorite meals to date.

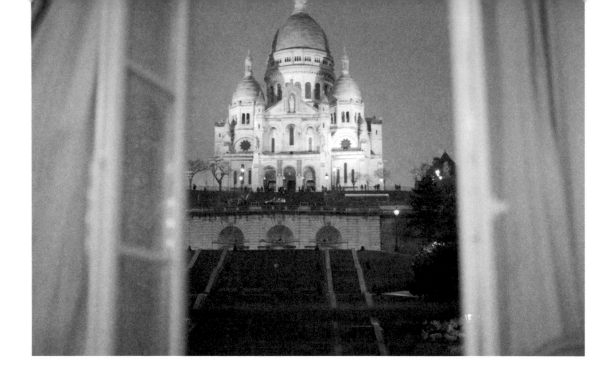

Sacré-Cœur

The most beautiful church in Paris, it also showcases some of the most picturesque views of the City of Lights. You can take the funicular up using a Metro ticket, or burn off your morning pastries with a walk up the many, many steps. Once there, meander through the busy tourist streets a few blocks away and find the mini village within a village.

Espace Dalí
11, Rue Poulbot

One of my favorite artists is Salvadore Dalí, whom Adrien Brody so perfectly portrayed in a brief but memorable scene in *Midnight in Paris*. This small museum is easy to explore and a must stop for lovers of Surrealism and Cubist art.

Musée de Montmartre
12, Rue Cortot

The oldest building in Montmartre, it has housed the studios of many artists, including Renoir, Valadon, Émile Bernard, and others. The artwork on display shares the colorful history of Montmartre, including the Moulin Rouge, Le Chat Noir, and the Clos Vineyard. Montmartre girls enjoy walking through the exhibitions, which change regularly. The lovely gardens have been transformed to appear as they did in Renoir's paintings and offer surreal views of the vineyard and the rooftops of Paris.

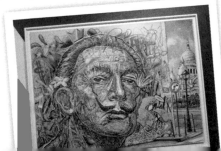

Le Grand 8
8, Rue Lamarck

With natural wines and simple cooking, this low-key neighborhood bistro is a favorite of local residents, chefs, and winemakers. Their Sunday night parties, where other chefs and neighborhood friends stay late for good wines and good conversation, are legendary.

Place du Tertre

This quaint square located a few blocks behind Sacré-Cœur is filled with artists selling original paintings and illustrations, and a few doing portraits or caricatures of visitors. It can be crowded at times but always worth a quick walk-through to see the original and affordable artwork for sale. There is one artist in particular whom I have purchased four paintings on canvas from over the past ten years and whose work I am building a nice collection of. A couple of the cafés on the square have canopied areas to dine outside, with heaters during colder months. It won't be an amazing meal, but if you need a quick croque monsieur or roast chicken, it's a relaxing place to sit and people watch.

Clos Montmartre Vineyard

One of the many hidden gems in Montmartre, the vineyard produces twenty-seven varieties of wine. Grapes are picked and fermented in the cellar of Montmartre's town hall. Each October the vineyard hosts a five-day harvest celebration, Fête des Vendanges. Montmartre woman love to join the fun of this very Parisian and neighborhood affair. Enjoy musical parades, dancers, concerts, and fireworks in the evening.

La Maison Rose
2, Rue de l'Abreuvoir

This lovely pink bistro is decorated with painted flowers and vines up the walls. You may have seen a photo of the café flow through your Pinterest feed many times.

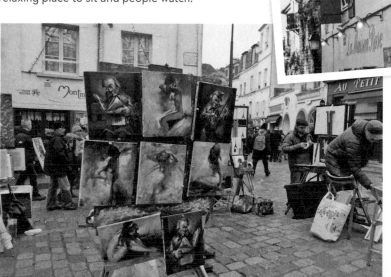

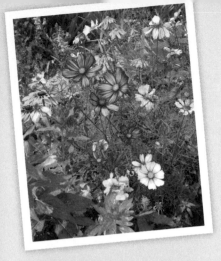

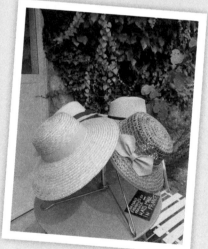

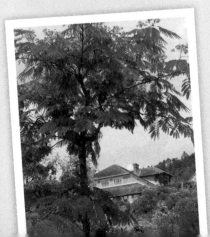

MONET'S GIVERNY

At the start of each spring season, Montmartre women crave inspiration. Not that Paris winters are as frigid as in New York, but after months of dreary gray skies, one needs a little pick-me-up. A quick cure for the winter blues is a day trip to Monet's garden and a walk through the village of Giverny. About an hour from Paris by train, the Montmartre girl will go with friends or sometimes alone with a novel to read in the gardens.

She brings along a straw hat to protect her skin from the sun, and a snack or maybe even full picnic fare. She'll first arrive at the train station in Vernon. When the weather's just right, she rents a bicycle rather than take the bus. It's about a forty-five-minute bike ride through the small town and over the river Seine to Giverny.

Wandering through the row upon row of flowers all mixed together in perfect harmony is an uplifting and enchanting experience. Her spirit blossoms with each step. As she walks past the garden and along the path to the water lilies, she remembers why she loves and craves this floral haven each year.

The Montmartre girl knows which flowers are in bloom each month and doesn't mind still chilly weather in April for a visit with the tulips and cherry blossoms. May boasts the hanging wisteria, which surround her with beautiful blooms as she ambles through the grounds under walkways and covered bridges. She'll skip the trip during summer months, when it's overrun with a surplus of tourists, and return again for one last trip in mid-September to catch a glimpse of the dahlias and rudbeckias before they disappear for the winter.

Not far from Monet's retreat are some adorable cafés and shops selling locally made soaps, beauty products, and floral souvenirs. There are also a couple of bed-and-breakfasts, which would be perfect for staying the night in order to view the flowers on an early Spring morning.

A seasonal guide to the flowers:

April: Tulips, Hyacinths, Daisies, Forget-Me-Nots, Cherry Blossoms

May: Azaleas, Irises, Wisteria, Wallflowers, Peonies, Daisies

September: Dahlias, Asters, Rudbeckias

Fondation Claude Monet Residence Museum and Gardens
84, Rue Claude Monet, 27620 Giverny

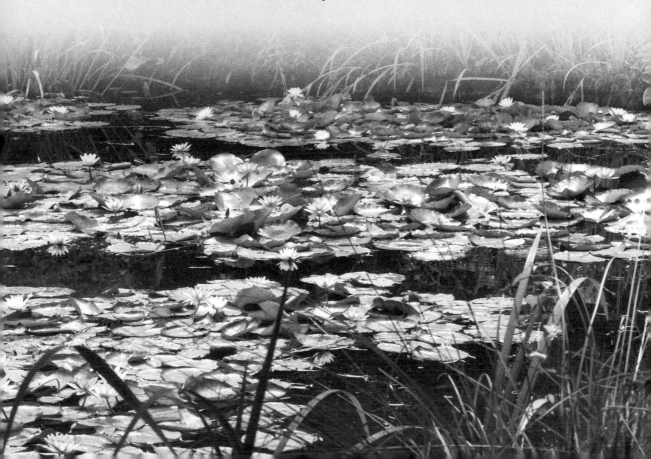

Le Passe-Muraille
Rue Norvins near Place Marcel Ayme

The *Passe-Muraille* sculpture on rue Norvins is based on a short story by Marcel Ayme about a man who could walk through walls. It's just another fun and quirky gem in this artistic village.

Hotel Particulier Montmartre
23, Avenue Junot

Hidden on the hills of Montmartre and down a secret passage, the hotel has a serene secret garden with a very romantic and private bar. The Montmartre woman enjoys going with her beau to enjoy a cocktail and perhaps play a game of chess. You don't have to be staying in the hotel to enjoy the bar, but you must make a reservation.

Fromagerie Chez Virginie
54, Rue de Damrémont

Here you can find another form of art in Montmartre—the art of cheese making. Virginie exclusively sells raw-milk cheeses in her family's charming shop, which is filled with mountains of cheese, crackers, meats, and wine. Sign up for a private or group cheese and wine tasting and visit the cellar where Virginie is aging and curing dozens of types of goat cheese to ripened perfection. This is a Montmartre girl's favorite stop before heading out to a picnic with friends.

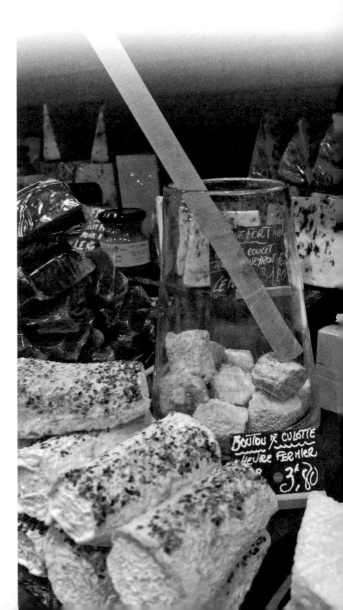

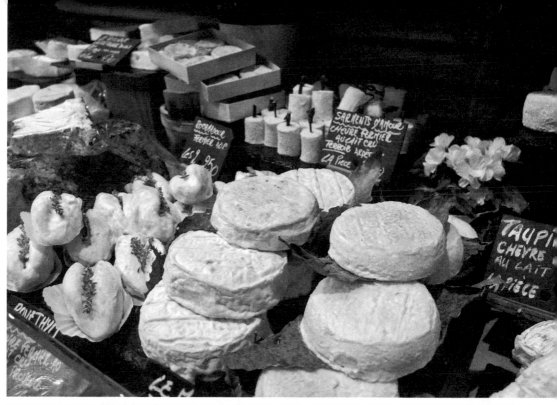

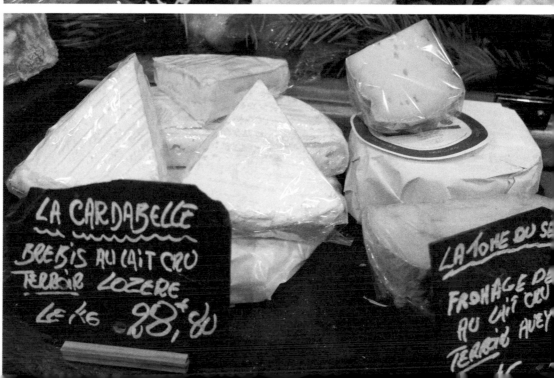

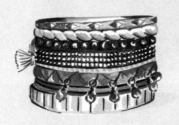

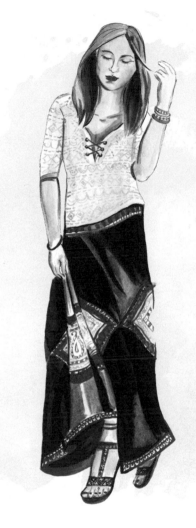

CHAPTER 8
CANAL SAINT-MARTIN

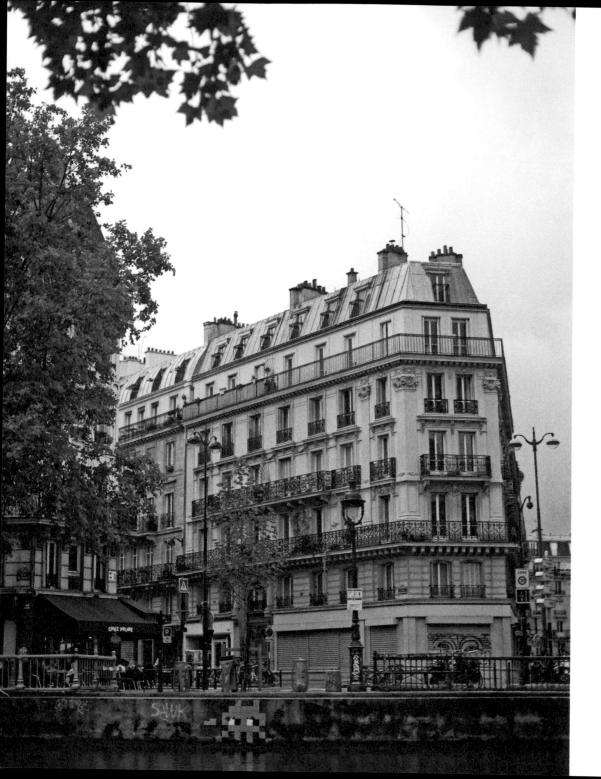

id you ever notice that Amélie (played by Audrey Tautou in the Jean-Pierre Jeunet film) didn't quite fit in in Montmartre? Her quirky behavior and bohemian spirit seemed out of place. But when skipping rocks on Canal Saint-Martin things just seemed to click for her. My friends and I were discussing this over lunch at La Verre Volé one day, and one of my Parisian girlfriends quickly pointed out that it's because Amélie carries inside her the true spirit of a Canal Saint-Martin girl. Just like that, it makes so much more sense to me now!

There's something mysterious about the Canal Saint-Martin girl. Turn a corner at rue de Lancry and see her carefree spirit wandering along the canal, deep in thought. She must be imagining the new pieces she'll create for her upcoming art opening. She's likely wearing a tiered cotton maxiskirt; a mix of wood, metal, and woven colored bangles; and flat beaded sandals tied around her ankle. She's 100 percent bohemian head to toe, inside and out.

Not necessarily a vegetarian, she nonetheless enjoys lunch at Sol Semilla, a tiny vegan café with healthy dishes and an assortment of powders and vitamins made from superfoods found in Peru. Le Comptoir Général is her gathering place for coffee, cocktails, or just a quiet afternoon reading a memoir or political biography. She likes to shop along the canal for kitschy housewares at Antoine et Lili, art books at Artazart, and tiny jewelry trinkets at Dante & Maria.

When her girlfriends who live in other neighborhoods are in the mood for outlet shopping, they visit her area for some of the best-stock shops without all the crowds. She tags along and occasionally finds something that fits her style, but usually she's just there for moral support, making sure they don't waste money shopping for items they don't actually need in their closets.

Often found picnicking on the canal, the Canal Saint-Martin girl also loves to congregate in the courtyard of her building with friends and neighbors for a summer soiree and hosts très casual dinner parties. Her home décor is boho Moroccan with interesting art books and magazines spread about her space.

Thanks to being an artist, she can get into any museum in Paris for free. She's up for any adventure and never tires of wandering her neighborhood or nearby Belleville to see the newest graffiti street art and space invaders that have popped up.

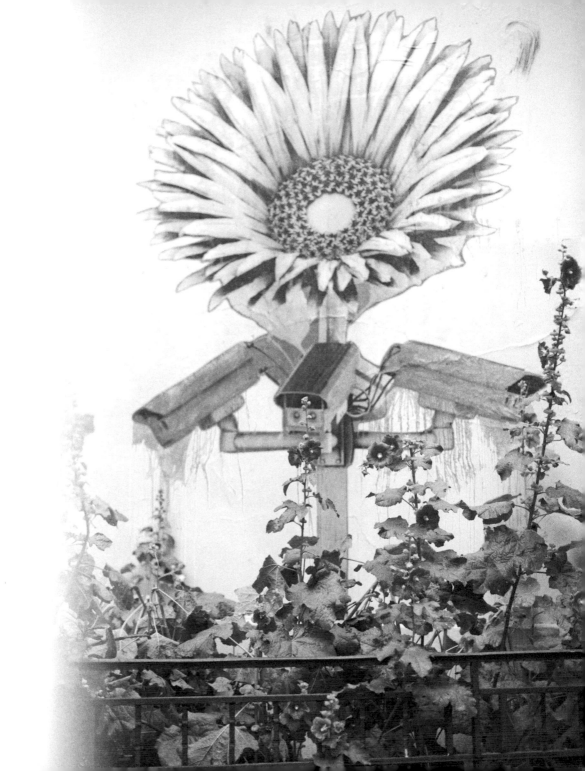

GET THE CANAL
SAINT-MARTIN LOOK

Without question, the number-one brand that captures the boho-chic lifestyle through their collections and marketing is Free People. Industry insiders and fashionistas alike anxiously await what the brand will unveil each season. I, of course, hold a soft spot for their catalogs, which are shot in Paris by Guy Aroch.

Put together head-to-toe boho-chic looks at the Free People boutiques and check their website regularly for special online exclusives: www.FreePeople.com.

To the Max

Maxidresses and skirts in all varieties—cotton, silk, tiered, pleated, flora, sheer layers, and more—line the Canal Saint-Martin's girl closet. You can find all styles at Free People.

Bangles

You can find bangles at so many boutiques, in a wide range of prices. The key is to mix it up with wood, metal, different colors, and a little beading (especially turquoise). Free People sells cool hand bracelets and armbands to add an extra-special touch to your boho-chic look.

Peasantry

Peasant tops with delicate cutouts and embellishments, and sheer camisole tops in both prints and solid colors, are paired with lace bandeau bras.

Beaded Sandals and Boho Bags

French collection Antik Batik has mastered the beaded sandal and boho printed bag. FreePeople.com carries a few of their pieces each season, with additional pieces to be found on Shopbop.

Straw Hats

Free People has an incredible assortment of hats in many styles: beanie, matador, fedora, top boater, wide-brim, and floppy. The indie brand Worth & Worth is another collection that offers true craftsmanship and beautiful hats. Some styles are even named after Parisian neighborhoods like Saint Germain. TropRouge's Christina Caradona collaborated with their design team to create the "Christina" wide-brimmed hat.

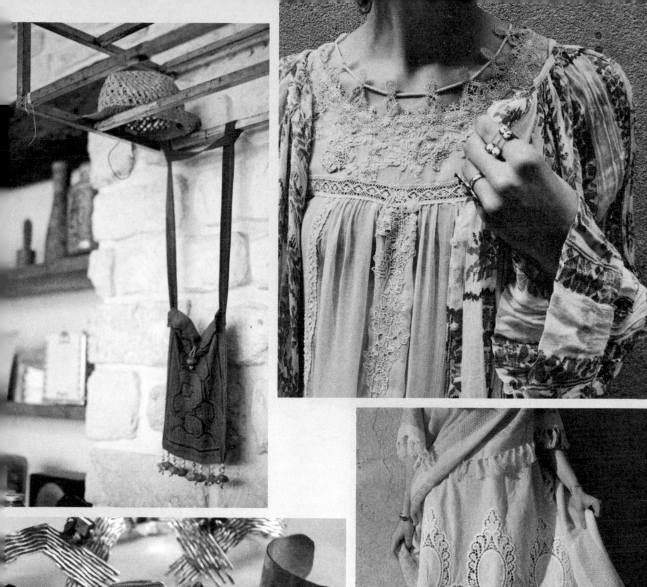
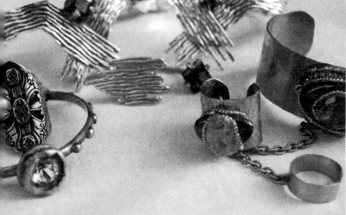
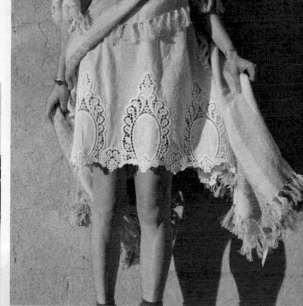

−*Carrie Harwood*, **FOUNDER OF WISHWISHWISH.NET**

Everything feels different in Paris. I know it sounds clichéd, but it really is the most romantic city in the world. After arriving on the Eurostar to Paris's Gare du Nord train station, I hop in a taxi. Driving to a hotel, I get to watch couples at cafés, old men on bikes with baguettes in the basket, and women walking tiny dogs—you almost don't mind being stuck in traffic! I can't help but stop by Pierre Hermé every time I'm in Paris—his macarons are undoubtably the best the city has to offer!

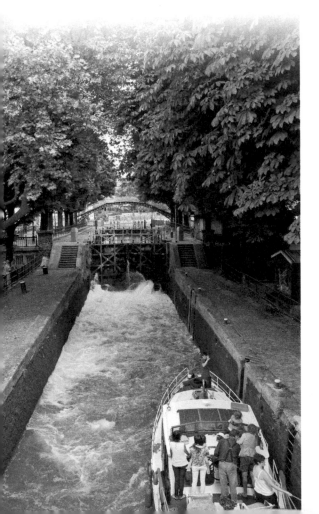

Gare Du Nord
18, Rue de Dunkerque

When Parisians want to head out to Northern France or London, they head to Gare du Nord. This stunning train station with glass roof was the location where Blair Waldorf said goodbye to Chuck Bass in an episode of *Gossip Girl*.

Canal Saint-Martin

There is a lot to see and do along the canal. In nice weather, Parisians pour in to picnic there. It's fun to watch the boats transfer from one level of water to the next. Book a boat tour to take you and friends on a sunset tour along the canal, but don't forget the wine!

Mon Oncle le Vigneron
71, Rue Rebeval

This gourmet grocery and wine bar serves dinner at a large communal table in the evening. You'll definitely want to make reservations a few days in advance for a chance at one of their cozy home-cooked meals.

Le Galopin
34, Rue Sainte-Marthe

This restaurant offers a daily menu of fresh seafood, vegetables, and meat dishes by one of the French *Top Chef* winners, Romain Tischenko. It's off the beaten path but always packed with Parisians.

Antoine & Lili
95, Quai de Valmy

Antoine & Lili is actually a series of boutiques selling quirky and eclectic clothing, accessories, and housewares. The multicolor pastel exteriors have made it a colorful and iconic part of the canal.

Bistro Bellet
84, Rue du Faubourg Saint-Denis

Enjoy traditional French classics with the finest and freshest ingredients near the Gare de L'Est train station. Girls in Canal Saint-Martin love that the kitchen is open until 11 p.m.

La Chambre aux Oiseaux
48, Rue Bichat

This is one of the Canal Saint-Martin girl's favorite locales for brunch with her friends. With an interior decorated like a vintage bedroom, she'll feel at home, but without having any dirty dishes to clean.

Pink Flamingo Pizza
67, Rue Bichat

This pizza shop has hot pizza and a signature hot-pink logo. You can eat there or have it delivered to picnic with friends on the canal. They give you a hot-pink balloon to hold on to so they can easily find you along the canal.

Hotel du Nord
102, Quai de Jemmapes

Expect to find a creative rock & roll crowd here. Nestled next to the canal, L'Hotel du Nord is often crowded, but serves delicious food in a lively atmosphere.

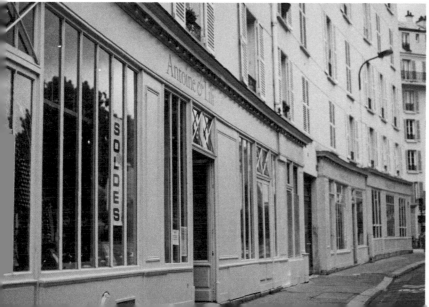
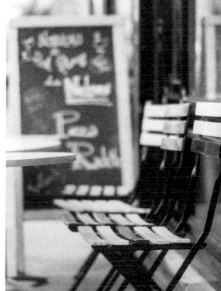

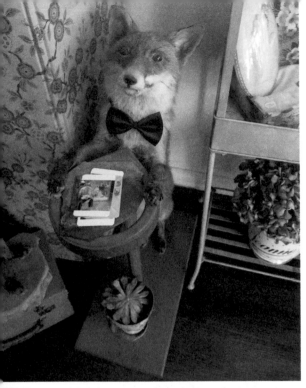

Dante & Maria
3, Rue de la Grange aux Belles

This is a favorite of Canal Saint-Martin girls looking for unique jewelry and trinkets by small independent French designers. They also sell mini toile scenes in vintage frames and embroidered with some R-rated remarks by local designer Marius a Paris. I already have a few in my collection.

Ten Belles
10, Rue de la Grange aux Belles

Having never been to Australia, I wasn't aware what a serious industry coffee was Down Under. That is until I first tried Ten Belles coffee. That's all I need to say.

Sol Semilla (Voy Alimento)
23, Rue des Vinaigriers

A healthy vegan café, perfect for lunch or a light afternoon snack. They also sell a line of vitamins and herbs made from plants from South America, in powder, pill, or liquid form. I've been a fan of the vitamins for years and always feel healthier when incorporating them into my daily routine.

The Sunken Chip!
39, Rue des Vinaigriers

This was the first fish-and-chips shop to open in Paris, which makes sense since you wouldn't usually think of eating those in Paris. When you combine fresh fish and French-fry sandwiches, it's really impossible to skip.

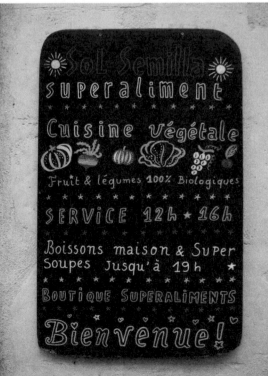

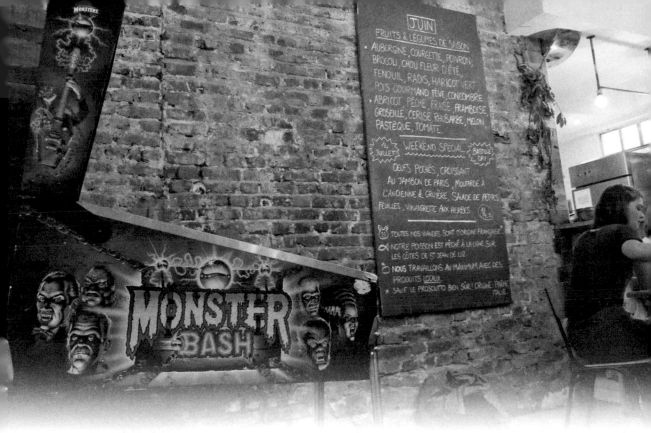

Holybelly
19, Rue Lucien Sampaix

The Canal Saint-Martin girl's local breakfast hangout. Opened by a team of cool Aussies, Holybelly serves delicious food day after day and some of the best coffee in Paris. It's a fun, low-key atmosphere with a pinball machine and a playlist of old-school pop.

Bob's Juice Bar
15, Rue Lucien Sampaix

This amazing vegan juice bar serves snacks and juices made on the spot with fresh fruits and vegetables. Canal Saint-Martin girls stay and eat in or sometimes grab a juice or smoothie to-go.

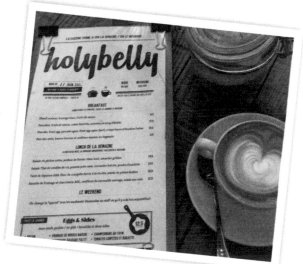

RACHEL KHOO'S LITTLE PARIS KITCHEN

My love of cooking goes beyond making favorite French dishes and also includes a love of reading cookbooks. It's a guilty pleasure to stay in bed late on a Sunday morning, flipping through and reading the stories behind each recipe to decide what I'll try to make next.

Two of my favorite French-inspired cookbooks are from Chef Rachel Khoo. I was never lucky enough to dine at her Little Paris Kitchen home restaurant, but I love re-creating the recipes from her cookbooks, *The Little Paris Kitchen* and *My Little French Kitchen*. I was thrilled (literally jumped for joy) when she agreed to let me include a recipe in this book. Like most famous Parisians (e.g., Marie Antoinette, Gertrude Stein, etc.), she's not actually French.

Originally from England, she has spent many years living in Paris and is a Parisian girl I aspire to be like. What I thought would be an impossible decision of selecting a recipe to include was made easy when I thought about which of her dishes I have made the most for my beau—her Poulet au Citron et Lavende (Lemon and Lavender Chicken). The blend of lemon and lavender not only tastes amazing but leaves a lovely aroma lingering in your kitchen.

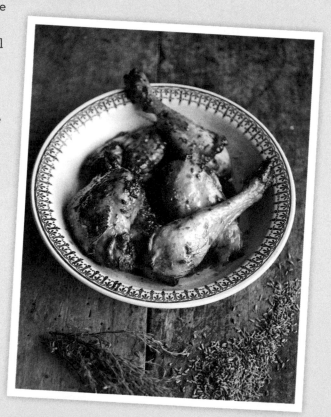

Poulet au Citron et Lavende (Lemon and Lavender Chicken)

From *The Little Paris Kitchen* by Rachel Khoo

The lavender fields in Provence are a spectacular sight, but if you can't make it to see them, I think that using a little lavender in your cooking is probably the next best thing. In moderation, lavender tastes delicious in both savory and sweet dishes, but don't use too much or they'll start tasting like Granny's soap. A crisp green salad and some boiled new potatoes are a great match for this summer dish.

For the marinade:

- 2 tablespoons dried lavender
- 4 tablespoons olive oil
- 4 tablespoons lavender honey or plain runny honey
- 2 sprigs thyme
- Finely grated zest and juice of 1 lemon
- 1 chicken, cut into 8 to 10 pieces
- Generous pinch of salt

To make the marinade: Crush the lavender using either a mortar and pestle or a rolling pin. Put the crushed lavender into a large bowl with the oil, honey, thyme, lemon zest, and juice. Mix well.

Place the chicken pieces into a large plastic container. Pour the marinade over the chicken and make sure all pieces are well coated. Cover and leave to marinate for 30 minutes (or up to 4 hours).

When you are ready to cook, preheat the oven to 400°F. Put the chicken and marinade into a roasting pan and sprinkle with salt. Roast the chicken for 45 minutes, turning the pieces over halfway. To check if the chicken is done, pierce the thickest part of the flesh with a skewer—the juices should run clear, not red or pink.

Serve the chicken with the cooking juices poured over and around.

Preparation time: 10 minutes

Resting time: 30 minutes to 4 hours

Cooking time: 45 minutes

Médecine Douce
10, Rue de Marseille

This jewelry store and designer workshop offers beautiful and dainty jewelry that you won't find everywhere else. Their chic gold bangles, necklaces, and earrings have become fashion must-haves.

Artazart
83, Quai de Valmy

Canal Saint-Martin girls shop at this design bookshop frequently for their impressive inventory of interior design, photography, painting, and modern-art books.

Le Verre Volé
67, Rue de Lancry

A great local dive that serves superb food for lunch, dinner, and even late night. This wine bar and restaurant is also a wine shop. Located only half a block from the canal, it's the perfect spot to pick up a bottle on your way to a picnic with friends.

Centre Commercial
2, Rue de Marseille

The Canal Saint-Martin girl likes to shop at this cool men's and women's concept boutique for up-and-coming collections not found all over Paris. They carry styles from one of my favorite shoe collections, Osborn, and while I don't purchase them here, since Osborn is based in the U.S., I love seeing this cool independent brand doing so well in Paris.

Café A
148, Rue du Faubourg Saint-Martin

When a Canal Saint-Martin girl needs a quiet place to work or just relax and be on her own, she heads to Café A. Housed in an old convent that has been converted into the Maison d'Architecture, it features a small bar and a few tables set up in a quiet garden.

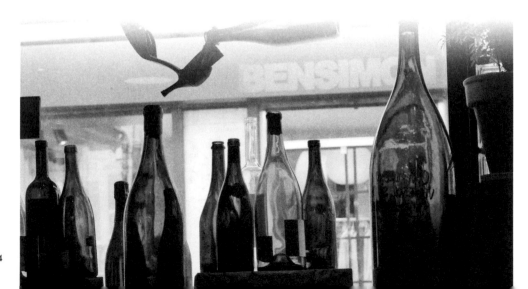

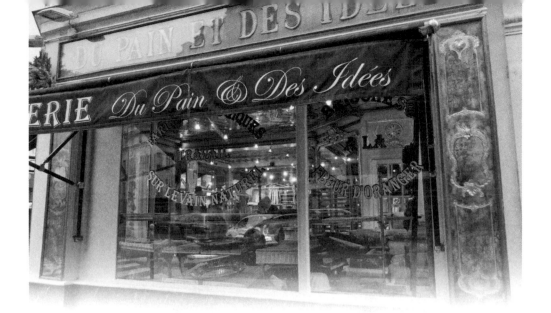

Du Pain et des Idées
34, Rue Yves Toudic

Located in one of Paris's last remaining boulangeries, Du Pain et des Idées has been brought back to life by baker Christophe Vasseur, who restored the beautiful 1880s interior to its glory. Because it's an authentic boulangerie, you won't find any macarons here but instead only specialty breads and puff pastries. Vasseur has perfected the classics like baguettes, pain au chocolate, and even "Les Escargots," a pinwheel-shaped pastry made of buttery dough with a variety of flavors such as cassis, praline, and my personal favorite, chocolate pistachio. You shouldn't leave without a full bag of goodies, especially his signature Pain des Amis, an incredible loaf of bread with a thick crunchy crust and soft nutty dough.

RUE DE MARSEILLE STOCK SHOPS

There are a few neighborhoods in Paris with multiple outlet shops. When you think of Canal Saint-Martin, you wouldn't expect to find any on your walk to the canal. But they're there and usually less crowded, making them much more enjoyable to shop at than others. While these collections aren't typically bohemian, the Canal Saint-Martin girl goes with girlfriends who do love these collections to help them make the best selections for their wardrobe.

MAJE, 4, Rue de Marseille

LES PETITES, 11, Rue de Marseille

CLAUDIE PIERLOT, 6, Rue de Marseille

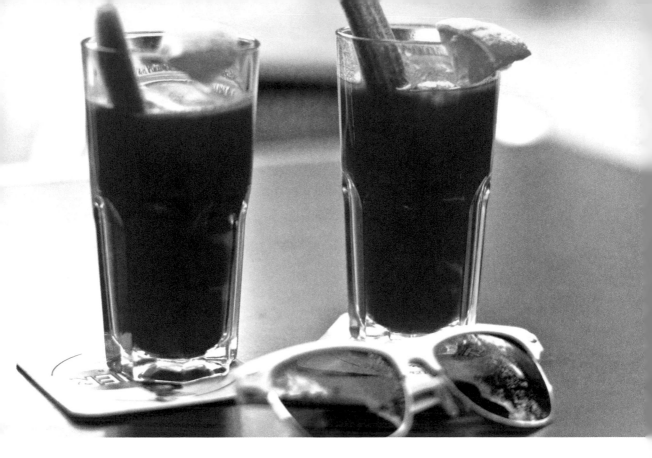

Chez Prune
71, Quai de Valmy

Located on a corner overlooking the canal,
this café is open till 2 a.m., a rare treat for
Parisians. Canal Saint-Martin girls love their
fantastic bloody Marys and mojitos.

La Tête dans les Olives
2, Rue Sainte-Marthe

This is the best olive oil shop in Paris. Since
they have just one table that seats five people,
be sure to make your reservations for dinner
far in advance. Your Sicilian meal starts with
an olive oil tasting, and your dinner menu will
be based on which fresh olives are in season.

Chapeau Melon
92, Rue Rébeval

This is a wine bar by day and a small
restaurant at night. There is typically one
seating per night, and they have a unique way
of serving the meal: they bring out all of the
dishes to everyone at the same time, so be
patient. It's an eclectic meal and absolutely
worth the wait.

Le Chateaubriand
129, Avenue Parmentier

There's no menu at this neo-bistro, which has been one of Paris's highest ranked restaurants on the "World's 50 Best Restaurants" list for quite a few years. Chef Inaki Aizpitarte and his team make fresh, minimal dishes based on each day's trip to the market. Canal Saint-Martin girls can't be bothered to make a reservation, so they stop by after 9 p.m. to eat at the bar or wait for a table during the second seating.

Le Dauphin
31, Avenue Parmentier

At this tapas bar a couple of doors down from Chateaubriand, Chef Aizpitarte has created a delicious menu of small plates. I can't eat there without ordering the whisky shrimp.

Le Bague de Kenza
106, Rue Saint-Maur

Towers of pastries fill this North African shop where you won't find any typical French pastries or creamy desserts. They bake up both sweet and savory, and most are made with ingredients from their native area: honey, almonds, and pistachios.

La Cave du Daron
140, Avenue Parmentier

A wine bar and shop across the street from Le Chateaubriand. It's the ideal spot to sip some wine while you await your tantalizing meal. With such great prices, I usually buy a bottle to bring home with me after dinner.

Aux Deux Amis
45, Rue Oberkampf

With a hot crowd and dive-bar setting, this modern bistro boasts a friendly staff and daily-changing menu. Large portions are perfect for sharing, but the grilled squid with squid ink risotto is so delicious you will want all to yourself.

Café Charbon
109, Rue Oberkampf

Not just a neighborhood bar but a neighborhood institution, this café has been open since the days of Napoléon III. DJs play cool music on the weekends, when the bar stays open till 4 a.m. Join the local hipsters on the terrace for lunch or dinner inside the Belle Epoque brasserie.

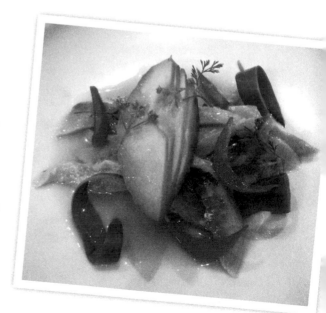

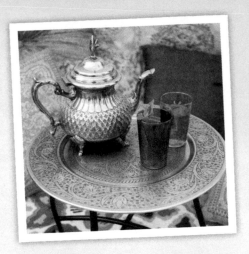

BOHO AT HOME

The bohemian girls of Canal Saint-Martin evoke a free spirit in all aspects of their life, including their entertaining style and home décor.

When they aren't hanging with friends on the canal, they are entertaining at home—usually a last-minute get-together and BYOB. Sometimes the Canal Saint-Martin girl cooks a casual feast, and other times it's a potluck meal; either way it's always eclectic.

She creates a boho oasis in her pied-à-terre, with an abundance of cozy pillows to create comfy seating areas. Her Moroccan-inspired décor is a mix of natural and jewel-tone colors. At dinner parties she serves Moroccan mint tea, phyllo pastries filled with lamb and chicken, vegetable kebabs, and couscous. Friends laugh, dance barefoot, smoke from the hookah, and share stories till the early morning hours.

While I love bohemian décor, it isn't something I want throughout my entire home. I do, however, love a bohemian backyard or rooftop deck. It becomes my dreamy oasis I can escape to without going too far.

Anthropologie and ABC Carpet & Home are two of my favorite stores for creating a chic bohemian hideaway. Mix patterns and colors, focusing a lot on jewel tones. Many of the items in the accompanying photos were purchased at Anthropologie, including the rug, and even bedroom curtains repurposed to create the perfect backdrop of my rooftop hideaway. Above all, don't forget lots of comfy pillows to lounge around on. These I found at World Market.

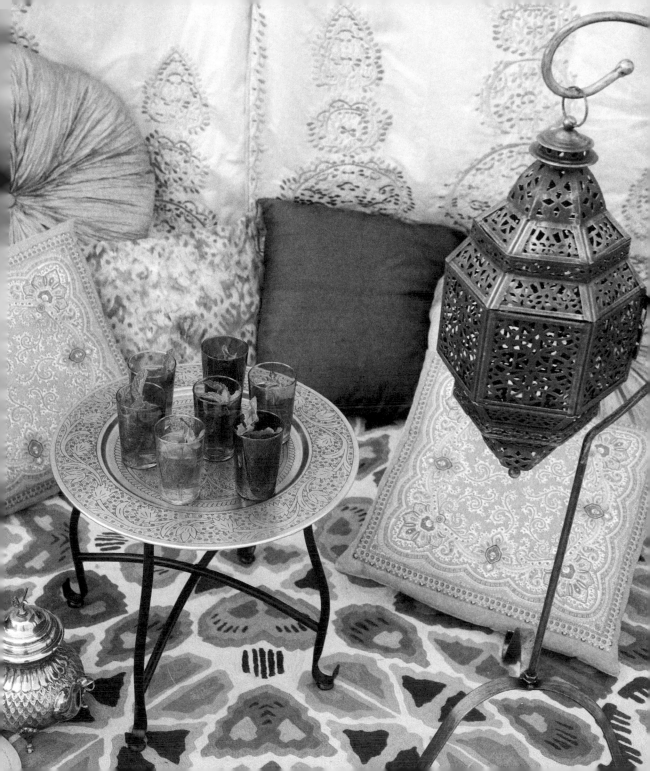

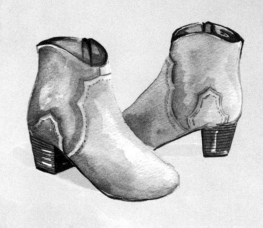

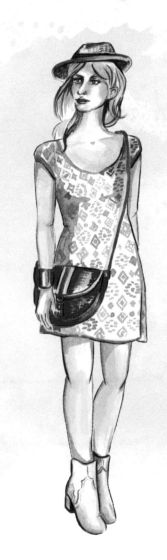

CHAPTER 9

BASTILLE

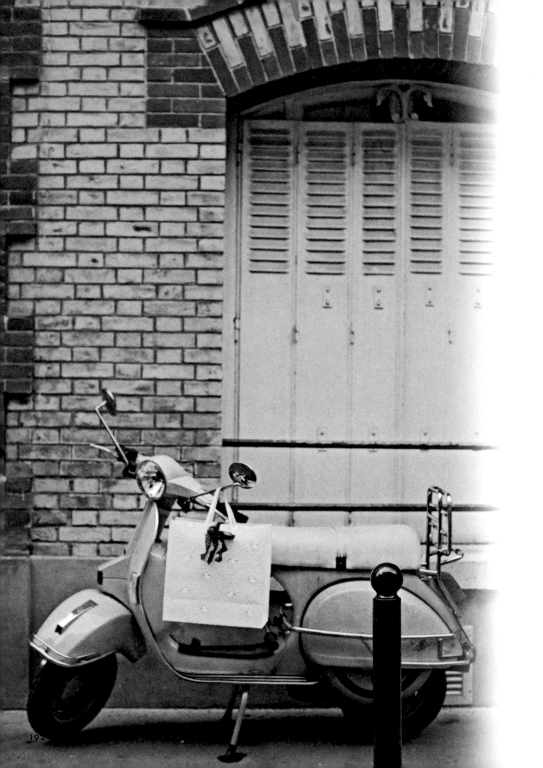

till central Paris but not the center of town, this arrondissement is much like the girl who lives here—a little edge with a rock 'n' roll spirit. The Bastille girl's look isn't as polished as that of the ladies in Trocadéro, but she still ties it all together and makes a strong statement. Isabel Marant's flagship on rue de Charonne perfectly defines this girl's flirty look of subtle but cool prints, year-round booties, and relaxed denim. She doesn't over-accessorize, and she picks one key piece to create her look around.

The Bastille, a mostly residential neighborhood, is a balanced mix of cultures. There's an easygoing vibe, which lures the Bastille girl to its many dive bars, wine bars, and indie concerts, and it has evolved into a go-to for many Parisians around town, while not attracting the tourists.

The Bastille girl definitely has bragging rights for living near many of the most talked about neo-bistros in the world, with young chefs who send out inventive, fresh farm-to-table dishes. Septime, Bones, and Yard are unanimous favorites. Where desserts are concerned, she has an eclectic mix of bakery options, with African pastries and the best madeleines in Paris.

When she's not dining out, she goes food shopping at one of Paris's best open food markets, Marche d'Aligre, where she can pick up fresh fruit, vegetables, and gourmet food items. Some Bastille girls even grow their own vegetables at a nearby greenhouse.

Place de la Bastille was the famous location where the French Revolution began and is celebrated on French National Day, also known as Bastille Day, on July 14. The aboveground park, La Promenade Plantée, is a favorite for an easygoing walk in the midst of the crowded streets of Paris and was the model for New York City's High Line Park.

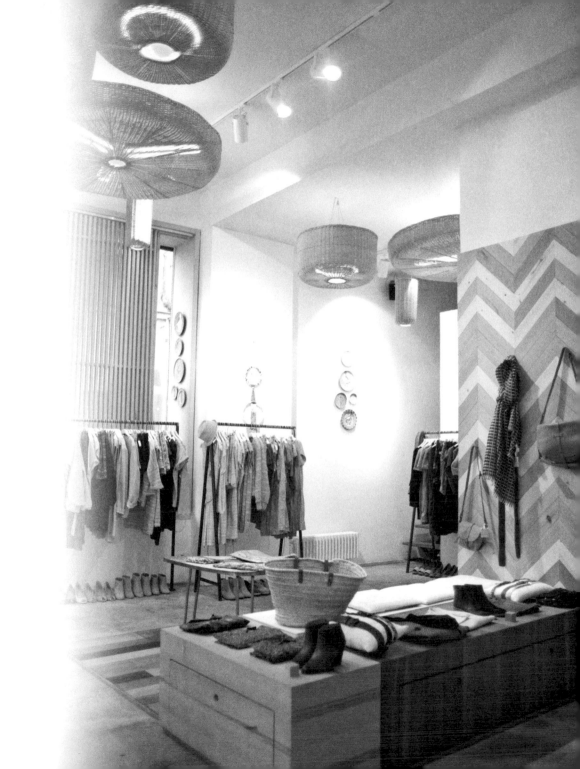

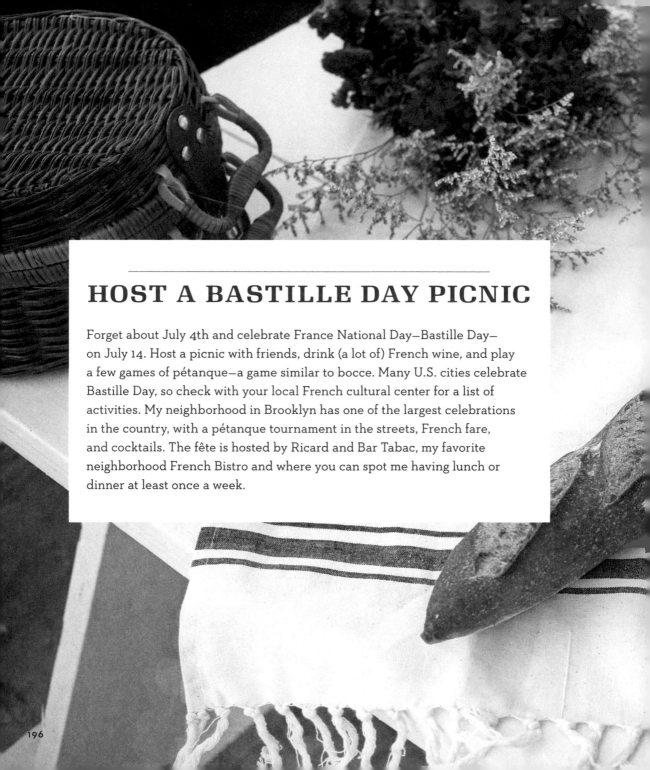

HOST A BASTILLE DAY PICNIC

Forget about July 4th and celebrate France National Day—Bastille Day—on July 14. Host a picnic with friends, drink (a lot of) French wine, and play a few games of pétanque—a game similar to bocce. Many U.S. cities celebrate Bastille Day, so check with your local French cultural center for a list of activities. My neighborhood in Brooklyn has one of the largest celebrations in the country, with a pétanque tournament in the streets, French fare, and cocktails. The fête is hosted by Ricard and Bar Tabac, my favorite neighborhood French Bistro and where you can spot me having lunch or dinner at least once a week.

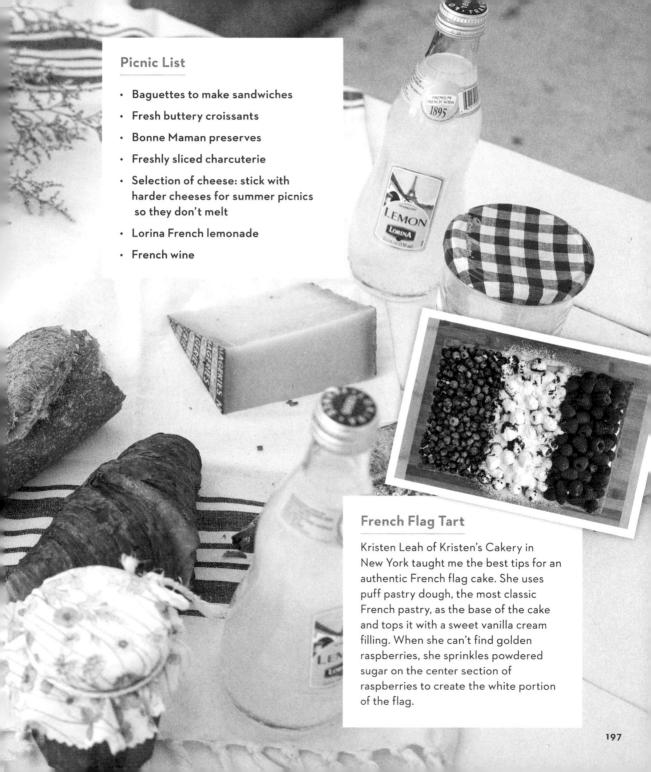

Picnic List

- Baguettes to make sandwiches
- Fresh buttery croissants
- Bonne Maman preserves
- Freshly sliced charcuterie
- Selection of cheese: stick with harder cheeses for summer picnics so they don't melt
- Lorina French lemonade
- French wine

French Flag Tart

Kristen Leah of Kristen's Cakery in New York taught me the best tips for an authentic French flag cake. She uses puff pastry dough, the most classic French pastry, as the base of the cake and tops it with a sweet vanilla cream filling. When she can't find golden raspberries, she sprinkles powdered sugar on the center section of raspberries to create the white portion of the flag.

Bubar
3, Rue des Tournelles

There is somewhat of a chaotic charm at this wine bar loved by local Bastille girls. They order tartines at the bar and sometimes bring in food from another location in the neighborhood. It's also one of the few wine bars in Paris that carries an assortment of wines from outside of France, such as wines from Chile, Argentina, and Spain.

La Promenade Plantée

Bastille girls love this park to relax, read a book, or just stroll through without having to deal with traffic. On the lower level, below the tranquil park, there are lanes to bike without traffic, and below, on the street level, are the Viaduc des Arts arcades with craft and artisanal shops. Ethan Hawke and Julie Delpy took a long walk through the park when they reconnected in *Before Sunset*.

She's Cake by Séphora
20, Avenue Ledru-Rollin

You might not think Parisians eat cheesecake, but with thirty unique flavors (a few that are even savory) at this cheesecake and tea salon, it's a fun change on occasion from the daily croissants and crème brûlée of everyday Parisian life.

Le Train Bleu
Gare de Lyon, Place Louis Armand

This magical Belle Epoque restaurant at the Gare du Lyon train station is decorated with incredible paintings, chandeliers, and art nouveau touches. Even when they aren't headed out of town, Bastille girls meet here for drinks or a meal in an opulent setting.

Le China
50, Rue de Charenton

Enter another time in this restaurant with its Shanghai-in-the-1930s kind of vibe. Franco-Asian fusion food is served in the upstairs and live music concerts take place in the basement.

Chez Habibi
44, Rue Traversière

One of the Bastille girl's favorite neighborhood wine bars, Chez Habibi makes her feel right at home, with eclectic vintage furniture and live music a few nights a week.

Sardegna a Tavola
1, Rue de Cotte

This Italian restaurant serves some of the freshest, most authentic Sardinian cuisine. The menu changes with each new season, but a few tasty staples are always available and are a must—including the clams in a spicy broth and the prawns with taglietelle. Bastille girls enjoy the pretty Mediterranean décor, which is a nice variation from their usual Parisian bistros lined with red banquettes.

Le Baron Rouge
1, Rue Théophile-Roussel

This wonderful wine bar has Parisians pouring out onto the sidewalk and using wine barrels as tables. Very eco-savvy Bastille girls will buy a green glass bottle and fill it with wine from the barrels to drink on the spot or bring home. They continue to bring back the bottles for a great price on wine refills. Grab some friends, a barrel, and enjoy an afternoon of wine and fresh oysters from around the corner at Marche d'Aligre.

Le Square Trousseau
1, Rue Antoine Vollon

The homemade foie gras takes the cake at this Belle Epoque café. Its late hours—it's open until 2 a.m.—and location on a quite square makes it a favorite of the locals.

Blé Sucré
7, Rue Antoine Vollon

Pastry chef Fabrice Le Bourdat left three-Michelin-starred Le Bristol to open his own patisserie known for many a great delicacy, including the best madeleines in Paris. During the holidays, he also makes edible tree ornaments, which are glazed a special way so they don't melt when hanging next to tree lights. Crack them open when you're taking down your tree and enjoy chocolate that will still taste fresh and have a hidden surprise inside.

Caffè dei Cioppi
159, Rue du Faubourg Saint-Antoine

Noted as the best trattoria in Paris and a favorite of Chef Jean-François Piège, this popular date spot for Bastille girls is located down a quiet alley and off the beaten path. Parisians know that the only way to get in to enjoy their red wine and sausage risotto, and other Italian delights, is with a reservation.

Le 6 Paul Bert
6, Rue Paul Bert

This is a Bastille girl's favorite for their prix-fixe lunch of modern and inventive tasting dishes. It's also one of my favorite lunch spots in the Bastille; I enjoy taking a peek at the chefs working quietly in the open kitchen while eagerly awaiting the arrival of my steak and endive.

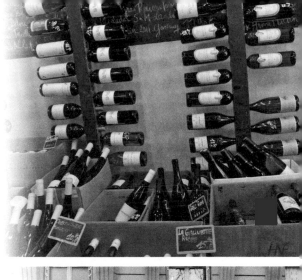
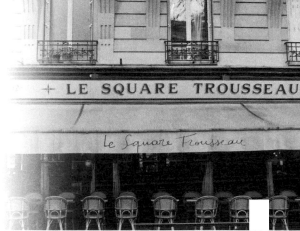
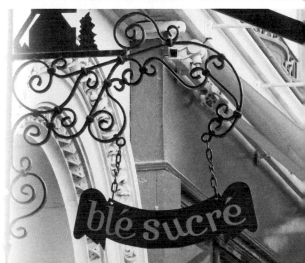

Le Marche D'Aligre
Place D'Aligre

This is one of the best food markets in Paris and a favorite of chefs, foodies, and the neighborhood locals. Serious collectors and dealers shop here for special vintage finds a few days a week.

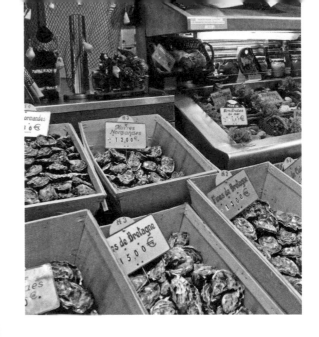

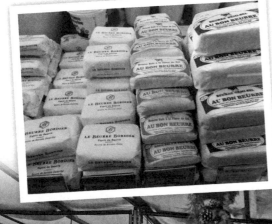

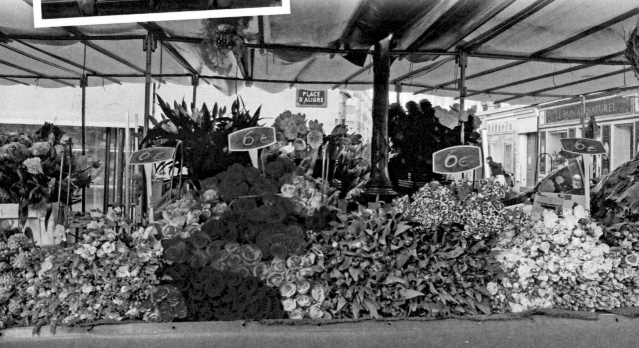

—Rachel Khoo, FOOD CREATIVE AND COOKBOOK AUTHOR

What I enjoy the most about shopping at outdoor food markets in France is that everyone does it and in Paris it is still very much part of everyday life. From your students, moms, young professionals to your French grandmothers, everyone shops at the market. The vendors, of course, have some fantastic stories and tips on how to cook the wonderful ingredients they are selling. Marche d'Aligre in the Bastille is one of Paris's most bustling markets, with both a covered and open part of the market, and on the weekend there's an antique market too. The range of ingredients is extensive and still very much at an accessible price.

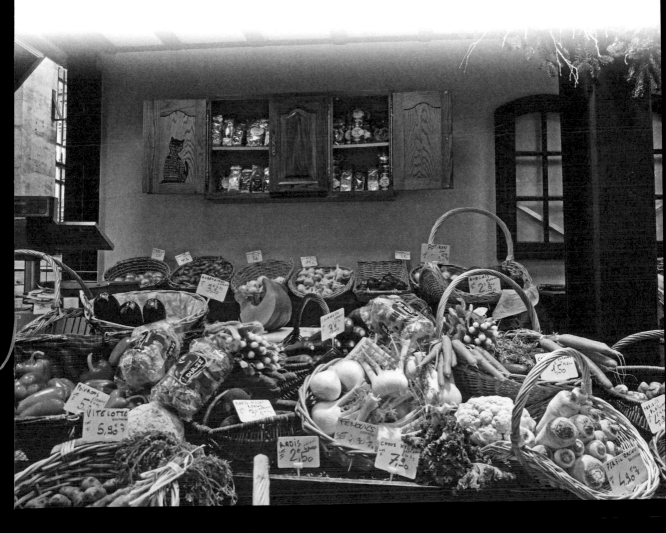

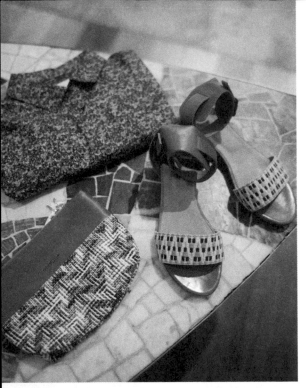

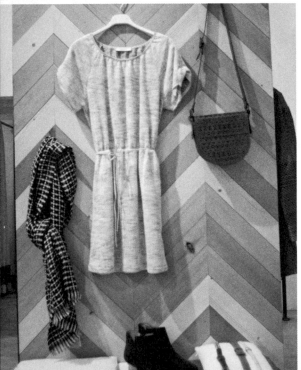

Le Bistrot Paul Bert
18, Rue Paul Bert

This cult-classic neighborhood bistro is consistently voted the best steak frites in Paris. Expect market-driven classics, crisp organic wines, and an incredible Paris-Brest for dessert.

L'Ecailler du Bistrot
22, Rue Paul Bert

Stop by for oysters so fresh, you'll think for a minute you're on the coast of Brittany. You'll find more than a dozen choices of briny, juicy mollusks, a variety of scallop dishes, and some crisp wine options to pair. When you're in the mood for a decadent seafood fest, go for the fruit de mer platter.

La Pâtisserie Cyril Lignac
24, Rue Paul Bert

Michelin-star chef Cyril Lignac is a new master at pastries and reinvents classics with a contemporary twist. Bastille girls stop in regularly, as the menu of sweets changes monthly.

Sessùn
34, Rue de Charonne

Sessùn is one of my favorite designer clothing lines and is still pretty unknown in the States. I almost didn't include it in the book in hopes to keep the secret. When I visit the boutique, I have the most difficult time choosing what to buy. Maybe one day I can splurge and pick up one of all of my favorites. What a dream.

Corner des Créateurs
24, Rue de Lappe

More than half of the pieces sold in this boutique are from independent French brands and up-and-coming designers. Pick up unique seasonal pieces to refresh your wardrobe without spending a fortune.

Isabel Marant
16, Rue de Charonne

Isabel Marant created the world of boho chic with her collection of slouchy trousers, off-the-shoulder sweaters, casual minidresses, and booties. Her collection is the uniform of girls in the Bastille, and her flagship on rue Charonne is their headquarters.

Oxyde
28, Rue de Charonne

Here you'll find a casual-cool collection of printed dresses and super-soft, easy-to-wear sweaters you will want in every color. It's a versatile collection that you could buy a dozen pieces from, mix and match them together, and always leave the house in a unique look.

Les Fleurs
6, Passage Josset

Down an almost secret street is this adorably girly home décor and accessory boutique. It's full of whimsical, magical items for your kitchen—and all other rooms in the house—that a Bastille girl doesn't *need* but of course wants. When I'm visiting Paris in December, I love selecting a new holiday ornament to bring home and add to my tree.

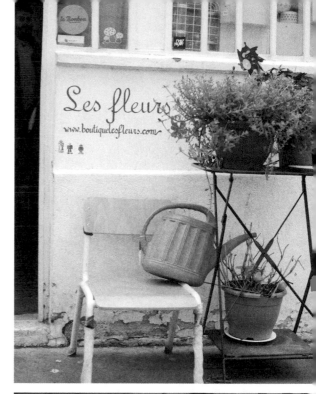

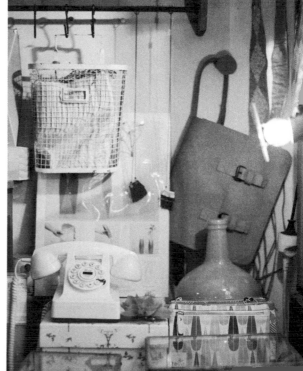

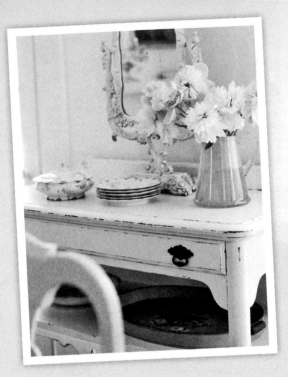

GIVE YOUR HOME THE FRENCH VINTAGE LOOK

French vintage home décor is a mix of elegance and rustic with distressed finishes. Buy vintage furniture and accessories at your local flea market or distress new pieces to give them that old French vintage look. Distressing furniture is a simple and inexpensive way to add a special touch to your décor. This style of furniture also mixes well with your contemporary pieces, so don't be afraid to mix it up. Great pieces to distress are wrought-iron beds, vanity sets, dressers, and nightstands, and you can accessorize a room with distressed mirrors, plates, and planters. Pieces with curved lines and carved details work best.

To create this look yourself, remove the original paint with coarse sandpaper and apply a coating of primer. Choose two paint colors: a darker one to be your base layer and a lighter shade to be the predominant color of the piece. Paint one coat of your darker shade and let it dry. Then paint one coat of your lighter shade. Once the top coat has dried, rub away small areas with a piece of steel wool or sandpaper to reveal bits of the bottom color. Use the sandpaper to create distressed spots in the corners, raised panels, and edges of the hardware. To protect your furniture, you can rub on a coat of clear furniture wax with a soft cloth. Skip that step and the furniture will look more distressed over time.

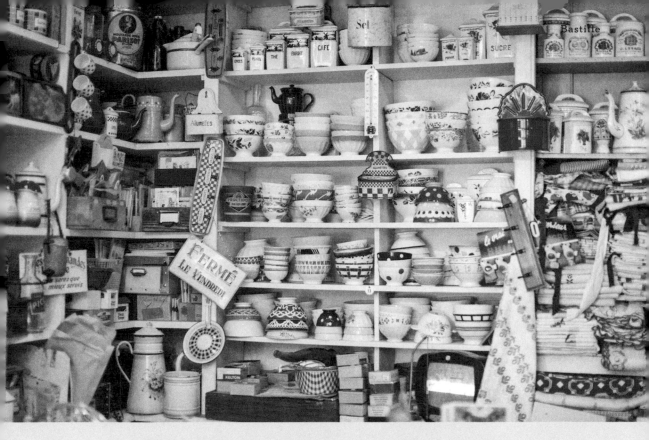

With kitchen accessories, non-matching pieces is the Parisian way, from plates and teacups to mismatched silverware and serving dishes. Flea markets, eBay, and Etsy are generally best for creating your own collection. In NYC, Fishs Eddy sells vintage dishes at a low price to mix and match. Or head to Anthropolgie, my favorite, for an assortment of unique and fun tableware. With so many wonderful items to choose from, I am never able to leave the store without at least one item from their home and kitchen section.

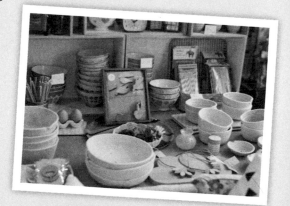

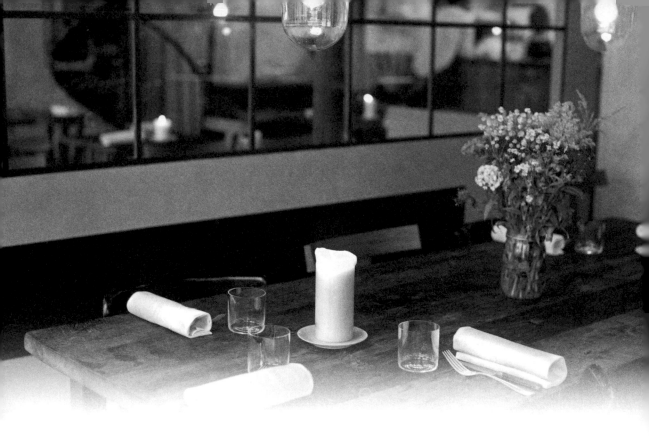

Septime
80, Rue De Charonne

Creative dishes in a casual farmhouse setting.
Tasting Chef Bertrand Grébaut's menu is a
truly special experience and an absolute must
when you're in Paris. That is if you can get a
reservation before Parisians snap them all up.
His ingredients are sourced from the best
farms in France, and he makes sure everything
is perfect, down to the last dash of salt. Even
the pork he serves is from pigs that are raised
on grass from fields with specific soil that
makes the flavor of their meat extra tender
and salty. Chef Grébaut's dishes are beautiful
to see, exciting to eat.

La Cave de Septime
3 Rue Basfroi

This tiny little wine bar is around the corner
and accompanies Chef Grébaut's restaurants.
You can buy a bottle to go, but with such
incredible house-smoked duck breast,
pancetta, and foie gras with smoked eel you
will change your mind and stay to pop the
cork on the spot.

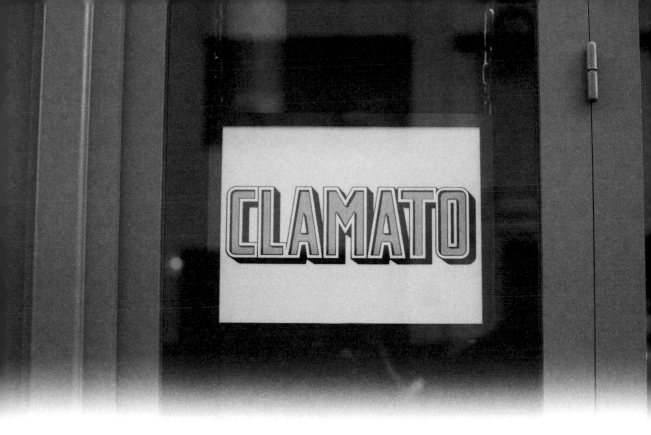

Clamato
80, Rue de Charonne

Chef Bertrand Grébaut, of Septime, also oversees this seafood and oyster bar, located just next door. Its cozy, bright décor is as welcoming as their oyster platters, crab fritters, and maple-syrup pie. They don't take reservations, so be prepared to wait patiently with the rest of the Bastille girls.

Come on Eileen
16–18, Rue des Taillandiers

This vintage store is the Bastille girl's favorite. It has three floors to keep her occupied for a while. She starts on the top floor and works her way down through racks of inexpensive 1970s dresses, an entire section of Converse arranged by color and size, and then to Chanel, Dior, and Hermés, in the designer section.

Gaëlle Barré
17, Rue Keller

Designer Gaëlle Barré doesn't follow the trends but always designs fun and flirty pieces each season. At the boutique, you'll find printed trims on solid shift dresses, ombré belted knit dresses, and the right accessories that are always perfect day or night.

Anne Willi
13, Rue Keller

Willi's understated collection of beautiful tunics in lightweight fabrics, reversible dresses, and lovely belted tweed jackets are timeless pieces you will keep in your wardrobe for a lifetime. It's hard to find in the United States but lucky for me there is a boutique around the corner from my apartment in Brooklyn.

Bones
43, Rue Godefroy Cavaignac

Aussie chef James Henry has been making a name for himself for his inventive dishes since his days at Au Passage. Henry's tasting menu is a magical mystery each night, with unique dishes cooked an endless number of ways. You could receive pickled, smoked, raw, and sautéed dishes all in the same meal. This hipster hangout of the Bastille has a bar up front serving craft beers, wine by the glass, and house-made charcuterie. The house-made duck just melts in your mouth!

Chez Sarah
18, Rue Jules-Vallès

This amazing vintage boutique is known for a selection of jewelry that spans decades. If you're at the Clingancourt flea market, look for their stall on Passage Lecuyer with a different but equally amazing selection of jewelry, accessories, and vintage trims and fabrics.

Le Square Gardette
24, Rue Saint Ambroise

From its exterior you would think this is just a typical Parisian café. But once inside you'll feel like you've been welcomed into the home of an eccentric Parisian with a million stories to share. If only the walls could talk! Vintage wallpaper, taxidermy animals, and quirky paintings cover the walls, and a piano in the corner topped with tattered back issues of *Le Figaro* creates the scene for this charming spot just perfect for lunch.

Le Perchoir
14, Rue Crespin du Gast

This "industrial chic" restaurant is topped with a dive-y rooftop bar that has jaw-dropping 360-degree views of Paris. It's the perfect location for a sunset gathering with friends. The scene among film-industry insiders and creatives gets crowded fast, so arrive early to skip the line and score a great table. If you stay for dinner, don't leave without an order of their seared tuna tapas.

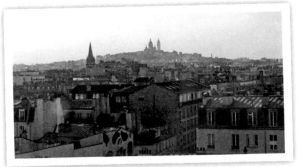

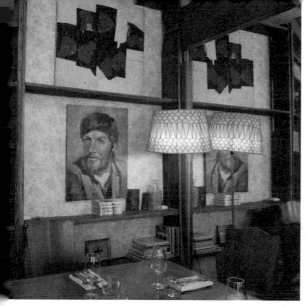

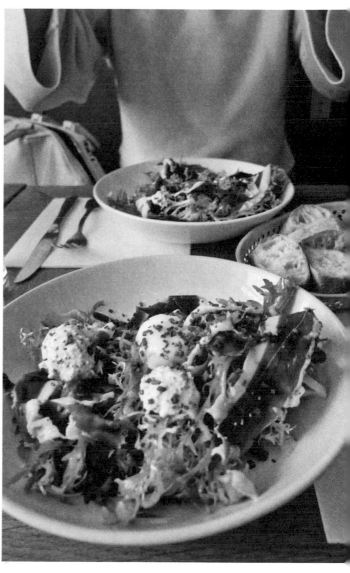

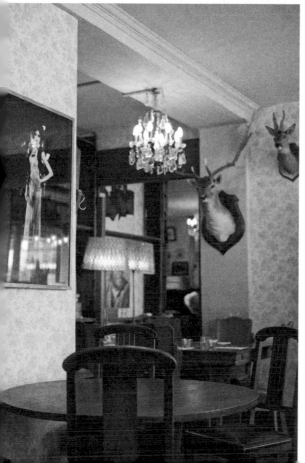

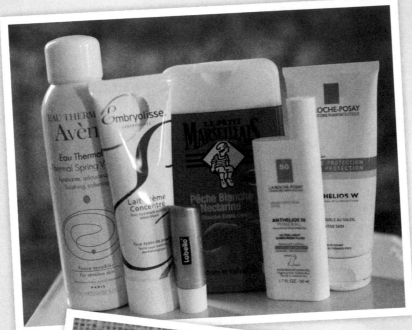

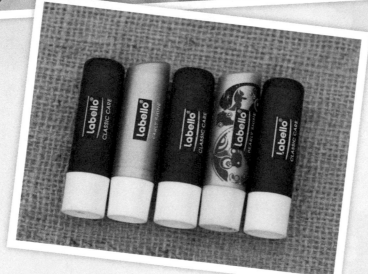

PHARMACY MUST-HAVES

French pharmacies are known for high-quality face and skin care products at affordable prices that are considerably better than U.S. pharmacy brands. Over the years I've tried several and narrowed them down to a short list of favorites that I stock up on each time I'm in Paris.

Embryolisse Lait-Crème Concentrate

This is an incredible multi-use product, which is very convenient when packing for a weekend trip. It can serve as a cleanser, primer, and a moisturizing mask.

La Roche-Posay Sunscreen

My fair skin loves to soak in the sun a bit too much, and I wear sunscreen on my face even in the winter. This lightweight formula goes on smooth and immediately gets absorbed into your skin. You never feel that greasy layer you get with most sunscreens.

Avene Thermal Spring Water

Spritz after using your cleanser or any time of day. You'll feel refreshed no matter how late you stayed out the night before and even after a long flight home from Paris.

Le Petit Marseillais

Sure, I was first attracted to these shower gels and creams because of their adorable packaging and delicious scents. But after discovering how hydrating they are for my skin, I am hooked. My favorite is the peach-and-white nectarine moisturizing body wash.

Labello Lip Balm

Founded in 1909, and technically not French (it's a German company), they produce the one item I never leave Paris without buying . . . and I usually buy three or four! You'll find at least one in my purse at all times.

A few of the above French pharmacy brands are now becoming more available in the U.S. (Check Duane Reade.) A few other brands that also produce great products include Vichy, Nuxe, and Bioderma. Some friends swear by the Bioderma makeup remover, but I'm just too obsessed with Bliss Fabulous Foaming Face Wash to switch.

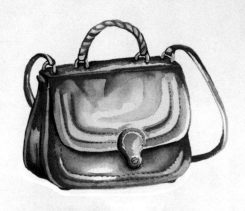

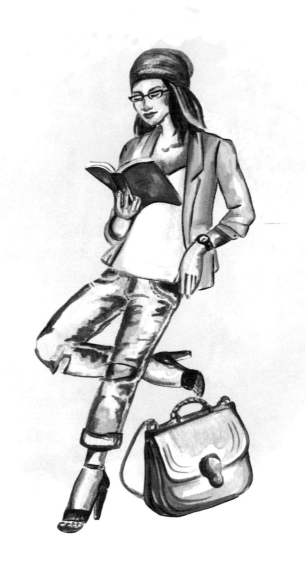

CHAPTER 10
LATIN QUARTER

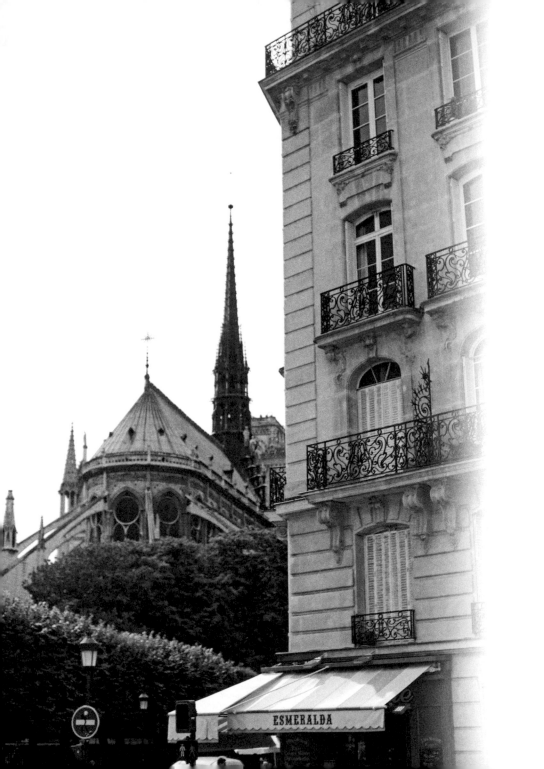

Piaris's literary land on the Left Bank is low-key and full of dreamers, thinkers, and philosophers. It's the arrondissement where students fall in love over philosophy, poetry, and baguettes.

The Latin Quarter girl is casual, and above all dresses comfortably—yet still remains chic (a Parisian girl characteristic). Her wardrobe consists of seasonal basics, tees, boyfriend jeans, and the perfect leather tote to carry her books, writing journals, and lunch to-go. She's just as happy sitting on a bench watching the world go by as she is at a bar with friends. The Latin Quarter girl goes on romantic walks at night—even by herself—crossing Paris's oldest bridge, Pont Neuf, into the bordering islands of Île Saint-Louis and Île de la Cité. During the day she spends time quietly reading and relaxing in the hidden parks not known by tourists. On Sunday mornings she enjoys walking through the peaceful Place Dauphine on her way to the bird and flower market, where she'll pick up a few new plants to put out on her windowsill. She spends free time at the Grand Mosque with a pot of Moroccan mint tea and a copy of her favorite French novel, *Bonjour Tristesse*. She rarely spends time shopping for clothing, but instead browses the used bookstores and art book shops on Boulevard Saint-Michel. She's become friends with the *bouquinistes* near her apartment and checks regularly for their latest assortment of vintage books.

Rue Mouffetard is her favorite market street for fresh produce and groceries, and she frequently runs into the same eccentric ladies who live in her neighborhood and have shopped the market for more than fifty years. On weeknights she'll meet friends at the tiny movie theaters on rue Champollion to watch a showing of a 1960s Fellini film or a Cary Grant feature. On her walk home, she daydreams about living in that era before smartphones and laptops.

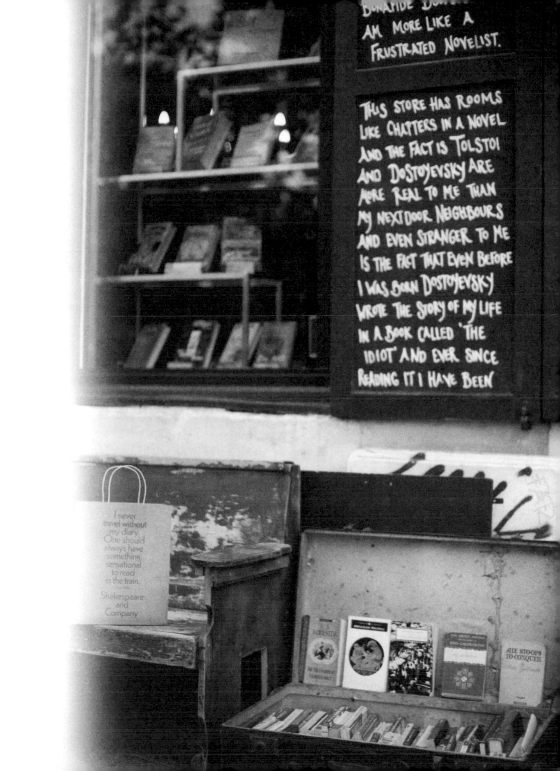

BONAFIDE BU~~~~
AM MORE LIKE A
FRUSTRATED NOVELIST.

THIS STORE HAS ROOMS
LIKE CHAPTERS IN A NOVEL
AND THE FACT IS TOLSTOI
AND DOSTOYEVSKY ARE
MORE REAL TO ME THAN
MY NEXT DOOR NEIGHBOURS
AND EVEN STRANGER TO ME
IS THE FACT THAT EVEN BEFORE
I WAS BORN DOSTOYEVSKY
WROTE THE STORY OF MY LIFE
IN A BOOK CALLED 'THE
IDIOT' AND EVER SINCE
READING IT I HAVE BEEN

I never
travel without
my diary.
One should
always have
something
sensational
to read
in the train.

Shakespeare
and
Company

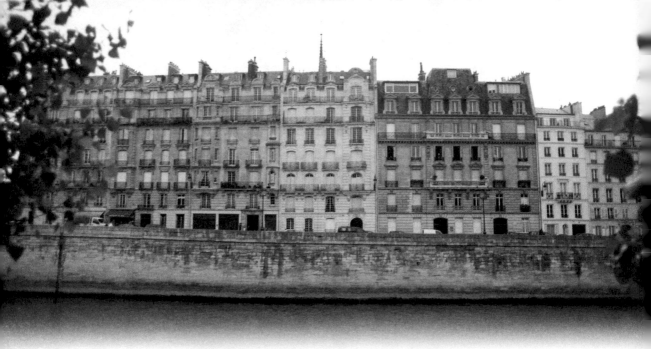

The Islands

The Latin Quarter borders two petite and very different islands, both with their own charms and hidden parks. The Île Saint-Louis is a residential village with many boutiques and places to eat and relax, while the Île de la Cité is full of office buildings that surround some of the most iconic monuments in Paris—Notre Dame, Sainte-Chapelle, and the Conciergerie.

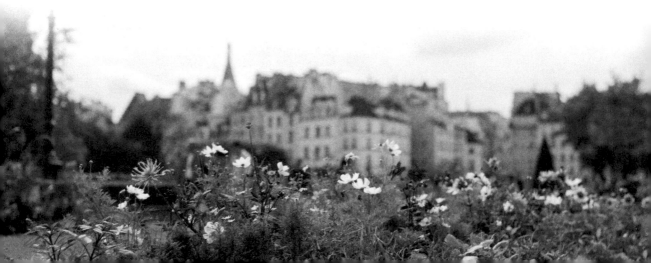

ÎLE SAINT-LOUIS

Square Bayre
At the Eastern Tip of Île Saint-Louis

More like a triangle than a square, this magical park is unknown to tourists and a favorite of Parisians. Latin Quarter girls love to go with their book of the moment and read in peace surrounded by both the Right and Left Banks of Paris.

Franc Pinot de l'Île Saint-Louis
1, Quai de Bourbon

At this favorite jazz bar of Parisians who like keeping away from the crowds, there is a restaurant upstairs and a jazz bar and lounge in the basement. Right on the water and away from the busy city streets, it boasts interesting décor, with mannequin hands and feet poking out from the walls and ceilings.

Berthillon
31, Rue Saint-Louis-en-l'Île

One of the best ice cream parlors, not just in Paris, but in the world. It's well worth the wait in line or braving the cold in the winter. Many other cafés on the island sell their ice cream, but getting it direct from the source is always extra special and worth the wait in line.

Claire de Rêve
35, Rue Saint-Louis-en-l'Île

This amazing puppet shop is owned by a little old man who looks a lot like Geppetto from *Pinocchio*.

La Cure Gourmande
55, Rue Saint-Louis-en-l'Île

This is my favorite location of this candy and chocolate shop found throughout Paris. Everything is just so pretty! Walls are lined with an array of chocolates (dark chocolate–covered almonds are my favorite), caramels, lollipops wrapped in a rainbow of pastels, and tins wrapped in bows featuring cute illustrations of children playing. It's like walking into a girly Willy Wonka Land. The adorable tins make great gifts and cute décor when you return home, to remind you of your travels to the sweet city of Paris.

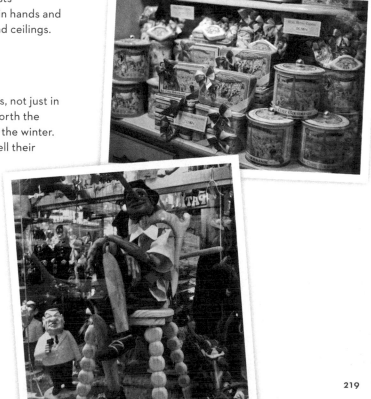

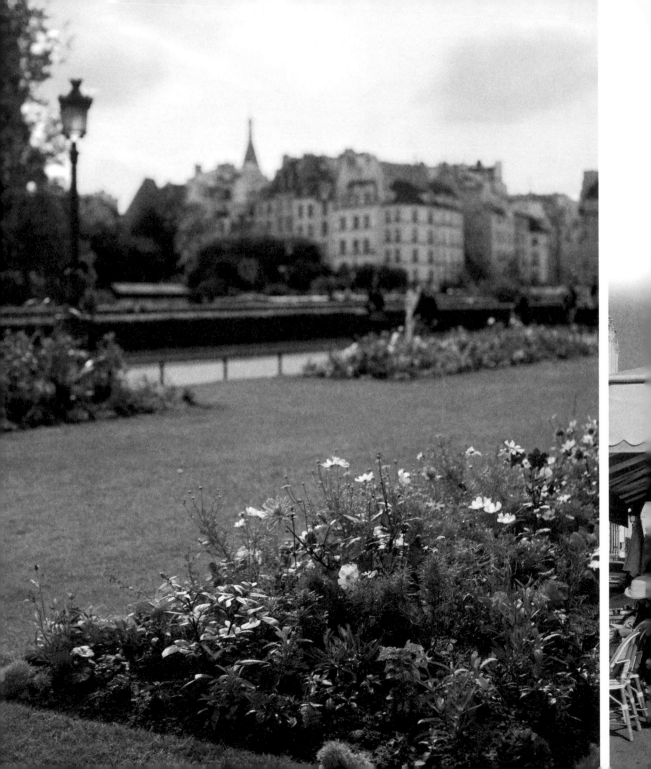

ÎLE DE LA CITÉ

Esméralda
2, Rue du Cloître Notre Dame

Overlooking the lovely gardens of Square Jean XXIII behind Notre Dame, this bar and brasserie is a nice space to be near the cathedral without being in the midst of tourist central.

Kilometre Zero

Search the ground just in front of the entrance of Notre Dame. When you see someone taking a photo of a bronze star, you've found it. It marks the "official center of the city" and the point where all distances in France are measured from.

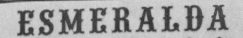

Marche aux Fleurs
Place Louis-Lépine

In the midst of office buildings is one of
the Latin Quarter girl's favorite places to
wander through in Paris—a daily flower
market that has been open since 1830. A
fragrant and colorful collection of orchids,
seasonal flowers, and plants has an even
better surprise on Sunday when it's
flooded with birds chirping the day away.

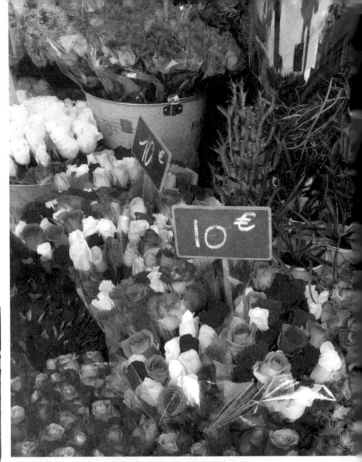

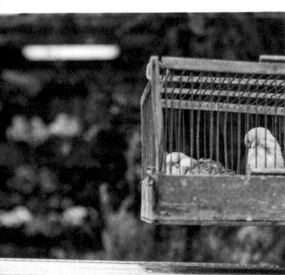

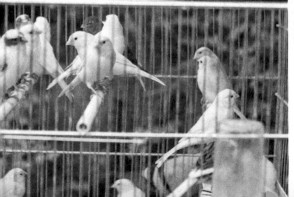

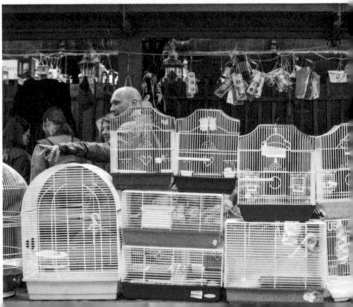

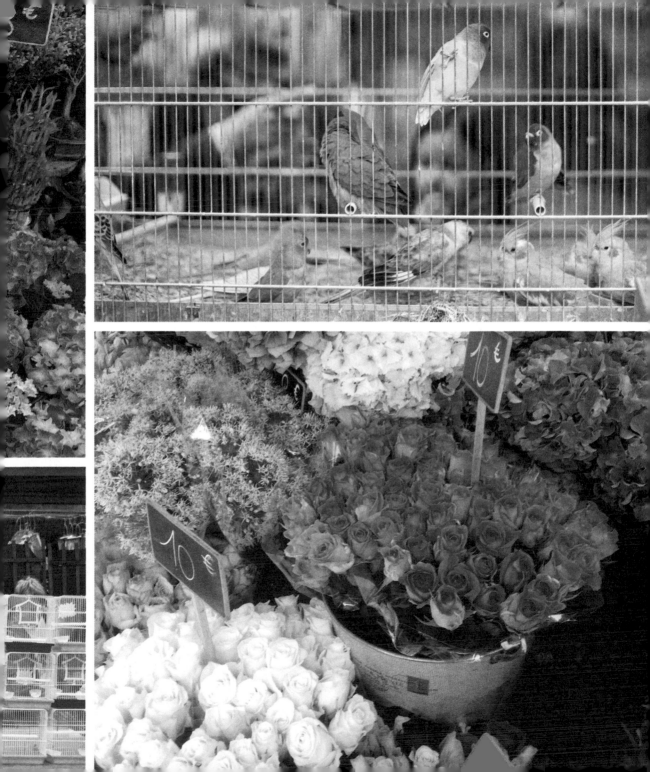

BONNE MAMAN JAM JARS . . . NOT JUST FOR YOUR JAM

I love fresh flowers. My favorites are roses, which I buy almost weekly from the neighborhood deli right near my apartment. They brighten any room, and just walking past them in the morning brings a smile. Sometimes I venture up to the Chelsea flower market for a mix of options and a fun reminder of the flower market on Paris's Île Saint-Louis. Instead of always putting the flowers in a cylinder vase, I like to mix things up and use wine bottles, a French Lorina lemonade bottle, empty glass candle jars, and my favorite, the French Bonne Maman jam jars.

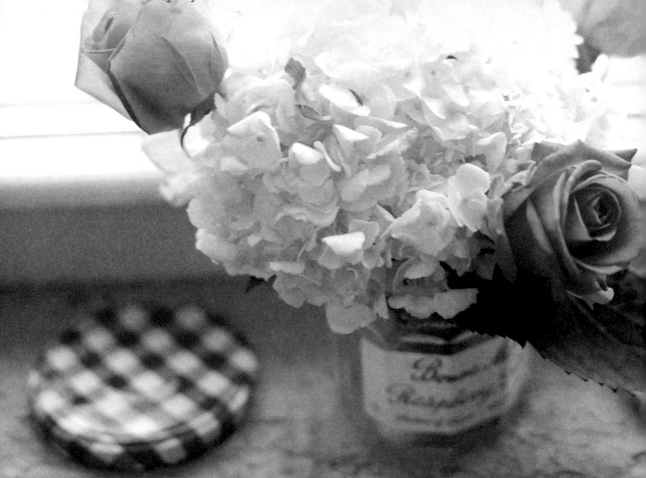

Hopefully by now you've enjoyed Bonne Maman jam or preserves. If not, *run* to your local grocery store and pick some up along with a few buttery croissants.

When I see the jars with their pretty font on the front and their gingham-colored lids, I'm reminded of living in Paris and seeing Bonne Maman preserves in all of my Parisian girlfriends' refrigerators. I love that they're now so easy to find in the U.S.

Once your jar is empty (which shouldn't take too long), you can reuse it for so many great things all around your home. Using the jars for floral arrangements adds a little touch of France in any room. Cut back your flower stems little by little to achieve the perfect height out of the jar.

The jars have many other uses. In the kitchen, use them to store spices, as utensil holders, or even to keep fresh herbs in water. If your bathroom is overrun by cotton balls, throw them in a jam jar and tighten the lid, or neatly display your lipsticks or makeup brushes there.

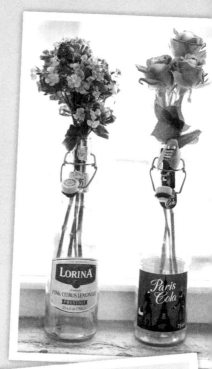

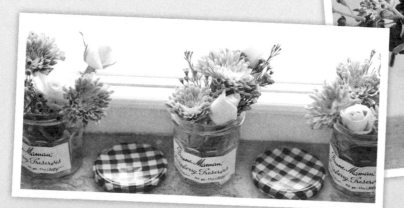

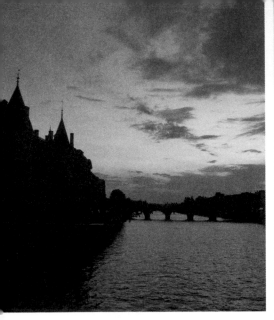
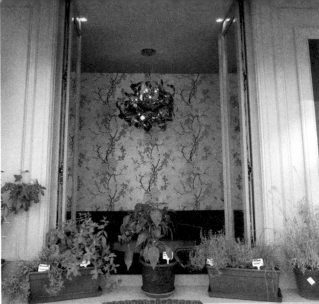

Conciergerie
2, Boulevard du Palais

Take in the magnificent architecture when you visit Paris's oldest remaining part of the Palais de la Cité. The stunning vaulted Gothic ceilings took my breath away the first time I visited, and still do each time I return. This former prison is where Marie Antoinette was held captive before she was killed. It's one of my favorite buildings in Paris; not only is the interior incredible, but the entire structure is awe-inspiring when you look at it in the evening from across the river Seine.

Place Dauphine

Located across from Pont Neuf is one of the most private and quietest squares in Paris. It was previously lined with seventeenth-century houses, but only two of the originals are still standing.

La Rose de France
24, Place Dauphine

With plush and cozy seating inside and a more casual feeling outside, this restaurant has great food and even greater dessert. Whether they stay for a meal or just afternoon tea, Latin Quarter girls always order the lavender crème brûlée.

Ma Salle à Manger
26, Place Dauphine

Nestled on the edge of the Place Dauphine, this tiny restaurant serves large, hearty portions of the delicious cuisine from the Basque country in southwest France.

Square du Vert-Galant
Pont Neuf

Walk down the steps on the Pont Neuf to find this romantic and tranquil spot, a beautiful tree-lined garden at the western tip of the island.

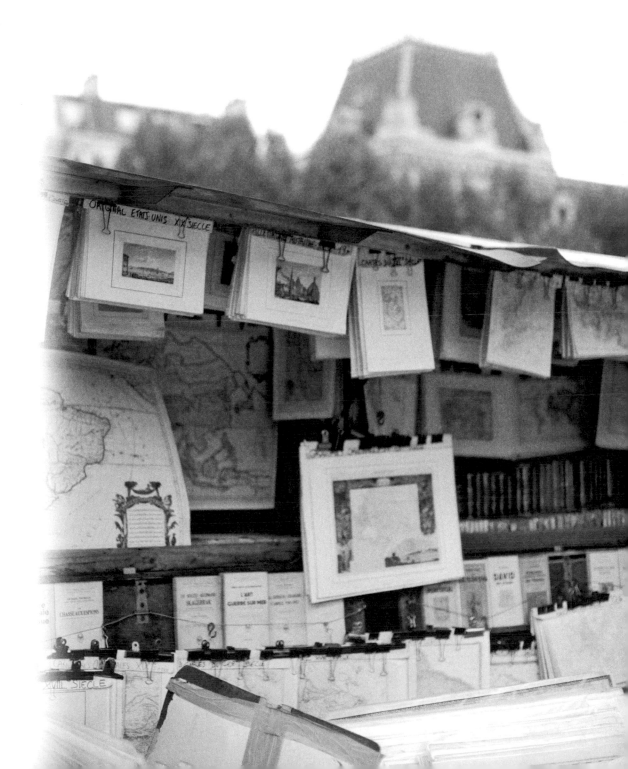

Now that we've wandered through the lovely islands, it's time to cross the Pont Saint-Michel bridge and enter the Latin Quarter girl's mainland....

Le Paradis du Fruit
2, Place du Saint-Michel

You'll find healthy fare, with a menu that is based around fruit, vegetables, and the freshest ingredients. Enjoy great salads, pita sandwiches, exotic fruit smoothies, and PLEASE save room for a chocolate fondue platters.

Etam Prêt-à-Porter
9, Boulevard Saint-Michel

This is the store Latin Quarter girls shop at for cute, inexpensive, and seasonal pieces. Find all the essentials, including swimwear, winter accessories, and loungewear.

Boulinier
20, Boulevard Saint-Michel

Stock up on new and used books, CDs, vinyl records, and DVDs. This shop has been a landmark in the Latin Quarter since 1845, and you can spot Latin Quarter girls browsing the aisles day and night.

Minelli
21, Boulevard Saint-Michel

With a focus on neutral tones, you won't find flashy styles at the Latin Quarter girl's favorite shoe store for on-trend and affordable styles each season.

Pâtisserie Viennoise
8, Rue le l'Ecole de Médecine

The Right Bank has Angelina, and the Latin Quarter girls of the Left Bank have this lovely café and pastry shop for incredible hot chocolate loaded with a mound of fresh whipped cream.

Shakespeare and Company
37, Rue de la Bûcherie

One of the most famous bookshops in the world. Much like the neighborhood, this shop was a favorite of Ernest Hemingway and James Joyce. An iconic and special shop overflowing with both new and vintage books in the English language, it's where Ethan Hawke's character signed books in the film *Before Sunset* and was a favorite of Owen Wilson's character in *Midnight in Paris*. The architecture of the shop is interesting—a maze of leaning shelves, secret cubbyholes, piles of books, old sofas, posters, and the occasional cat.

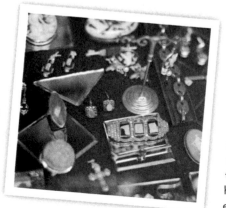

Les Metamorphosis
15, Rue du Petit Pond

A vintage jewelry boutique that I hold near and dear to my heart. I have a love for vintage rings and have purchased many from the quirky shop owner, who somehow remembers so much about the history of the pieces she sells. It's a history lesson and shopping excursion all in one.

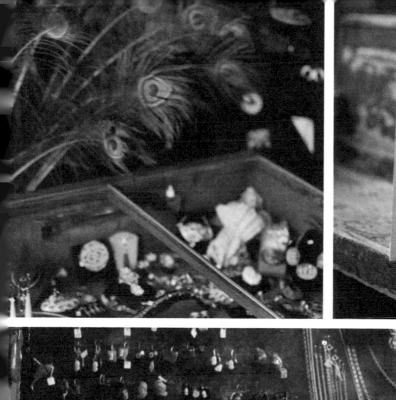
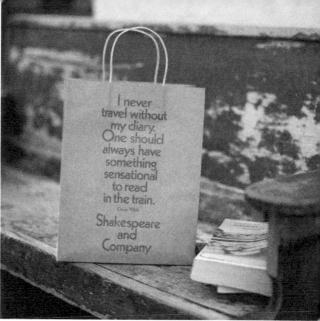

I never
travel without
my diary.
One should
always have
something
sensational
to read
in the train.
Oscar Wilde
Shakespeare
and
Company

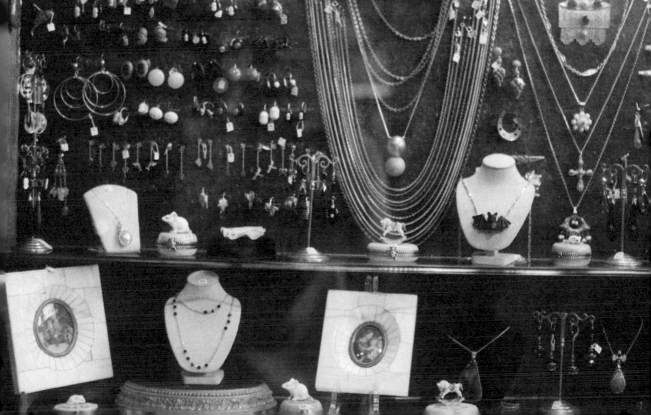

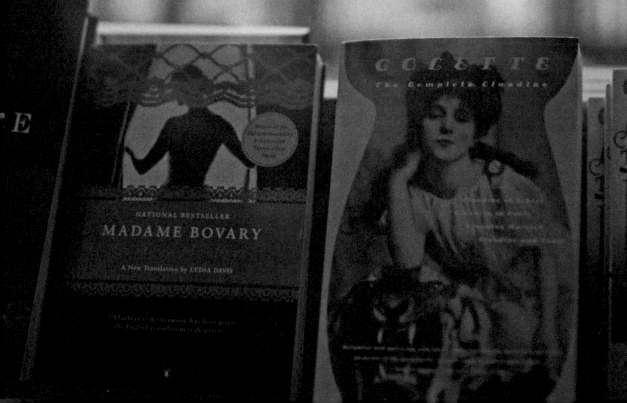

—*Christina Caradona,* **FOUNDER OF TROPROUGE.COM**

I was seven when we moved to Paris, and the first bookstore I ever went to was Shakespeare and Company. To help keep me from being homesick, my mom brought me there every Sunday and I was allowed to buy one book—as long as I'd finished the previous one. I'll never forget the first book I bought was *Alice in Wonderland.* I'm now living in New York but continue the tradition with my little brother and bring him to buy a book every time I go back to visit them in Paris.

READING PARIS

There are so many ways to learn about the lives and loves of the extraordinary French women of the past and present. Sure, we have the ever-entertaining films such as Sofia Coppola's *Marie Antoinette*, Woody Allen's magical love story to Paris, *Midnight in Paris*, and the eponymous film of Amélie's adventures through Montmartre. They all bring Paris to life in unique ways, and I continue to love and watch them over and over.

Like the students and philosophers who live in the Latin Quarter, I also love reading books set in Paris.

Get a bottle of wine, curl up on your couch, and transport yourself to the City of Lights with these literary gems . . .

Letters of Madame de Sévigné

This chic lady of court wrote eloquent letters, most to her daughter living in the South of France. Madame de Sévigné was quite the gossip, and she colorfully recounted the comings and goings of the French royalty and literary circles in the late 1600s.

A Moveable Feast

Hemingway's memoir chronicles his life in Paris in the 1920s with an animated description of life, love, food, and the restaurants Parisians still frequent.

Lunch in Paris

Elizabeth Bard's modern-day memoir shares her story of moving to Paris for love and the French recipes she has learned as part of her adventure of becoming Parisian.

Bonjour Tristesse

A French coming-of-age novel that was quite controversial in the 1960s and has since been reprinted in its original unedited form. Jean Seberg and Deborah Kerr brought the characters to life on the big screen.

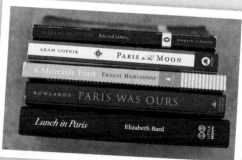

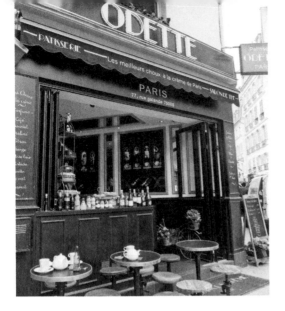

Salvador Dalí in the Latin Quarter
27, Rue Saint-Jacques

Stop at this address in the Latin Quarter and look up at the wall. You'll see a very cool sundial that was made by Salvador Dalí as a gift for friends who owned a shop here. It's these little bits of history and art floating around Paris that I find so special and fun to spot.

Sorbonne University

The Latin Quarter is home to several higher education institutions, but none more well known than Sorbonne University. The foundations of the campus date back to its original in the thirteenth century. Studies here are still dedicated to the Age of Enlightenment, focusing on literature, philosophy, languages, arts, humanities, and social sciences.

Odette
77, Rue Galande

This adorable art-deco bakery has a vintage bicycle perched out front and picture-perfect flowers on the upstairs windowsill. Sit and enjoy a pot of tea and a few choux a la crèmes topped with tiny candy hearts.

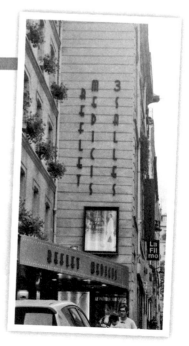

A PARISIAN NIGHT AT THE MOVIES

Watching greats like Audrey Hepburn, Cary Grant, Ingrid Bergman, and Jean Seberg bring to life different characters from past decades is magical. Watching them saunter through romantic towns in couture pieces from the 1950s or race through a souk in Marrakesh is even better when you're sitting in a tiny theater in Paris. The first time I walked onto the small and charming rue Champollion, I was delighted to discover three tiny art house cinemas. That afternoon I had the option of *La Dolce Vita* at Filmothèque or *Roman Holiday* at Le Champo. (Reflet Médicis was closed that day.) I made the logical choice of seeing both and enjoyed my evening of great film among the Parisians.

LE CHAMPO, 51, Rue des Écoles
REFLET MÉDICIS, 3, Rue Champollion
FILMOTHÈQUE, 9, Rue Champollion

Abou D'Abi Bazar
15, Rue Soufflot

Here you will find clothing and accessories in a mix of simple styles and eclectic prints. They carry collections from brands you may already know and from a few you'll find for the first time.

Les Papilles
30, Rue Gay Lussac

This wonderful gourmet shop and restaurant was opened by a former pastry chef at Le Bristol. Latin Quarter girls love the fun atmosphere and the chef's home-style menu, which changes daily. The shop sells gourmet items sourced from all over France.

Diptyque
34, Boulevard Saint-Germain

The luxury candles and room sprays made by Diptyque evoke scents of orange blossoms, black currant, green figs, and more. They have shops in the U.S., and their products are also available through major retailers such as Barneys, Neiman Marcus, and Nordstrom. Scent Explore 34 was created to capture the scent of the boutique—so you can re-create the experience of being in the store in your own home.

Nuba
36, Quai d'Austerlitz

Latin Quarter girls love the "make your own mojito" bar at this outdoor spot at the Cité de la Mode, located on the river Seine.

Le Petit Pontoise
9, Rue de Pontoise

A sign on the wall, written in French, reads, "We'll start cooking once you've ordered. Please be patient." Definitely not a bad thing, especially when they have dishes as tasty as the sea bass roasted in a vanilla sauce. I love that one of my favorite dishes in Paris can be found at such a simple and cozy bistro. Go for a late dinner to immerse yourself with Parisians and avoid tourists, who dine early evening.

Jardin Tino Rossi
Quai Saint-Bernard

During the day, Latin Quarter girls walk through the outdoor sculpture garden admiring the unique works by contemporary artists. From sunset to midnight during the summer months, you'll find them dancing the night away against the backdrop of the river Seine. There's music for just about any taste, with tango, salsa, swing, and even Brittany folk dances. (That's the Brittany Coast, not Britney Spears.)

Jardin des Plantes
57, Rue Cuvier

Usually overlooked by tourists, this lovely botanical garden is the largest in France. It spans twenty-eight acres, has multiple museums, and even a small zoo, which was first home to the royal animals of Versailles. Rows of cherry blossom trees in bloom in early spring, the Rose Garden with hundreds of fragrant species of roses flourishing in the summer, and the fields of dahlias in the fall make this a favorite of Parisian ladies almost any time of year.

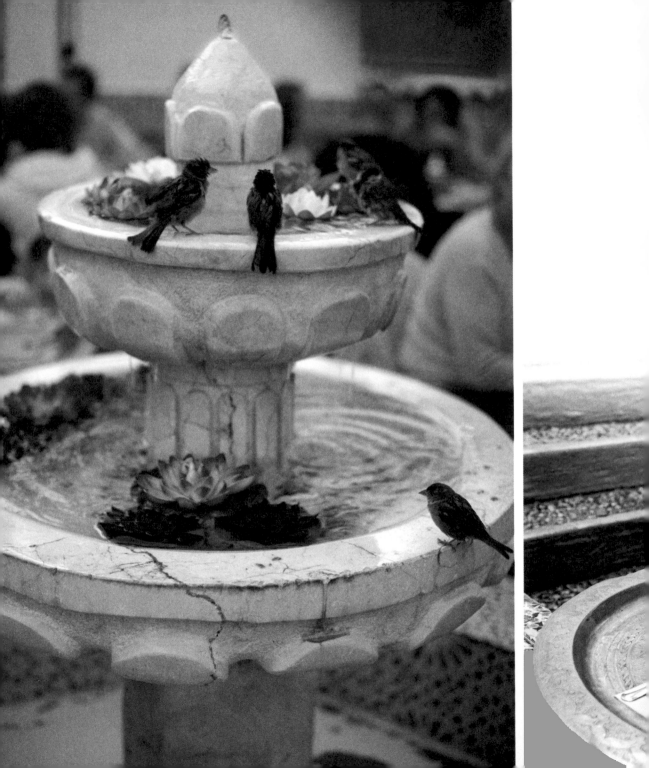

La Mosquée de Paris
Place du Puits-de-l'Ermite

Built in the 1920s, this is the largest mosque in France. Visit the fairy tale–like courtyard, where you can have mint tea and traditional Middle Eastern pastries. The *hamman* spa has a series of steam and shower rooms in a range of temperatures, a cold plunging pool if you need to cool off, and a beautiful fairy-tale setting. The spa is open on different days and time sessions for men and women, so be sure to check their online schedule in advance to prevent going on a men's-only day or time.

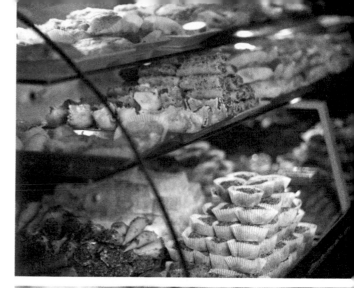

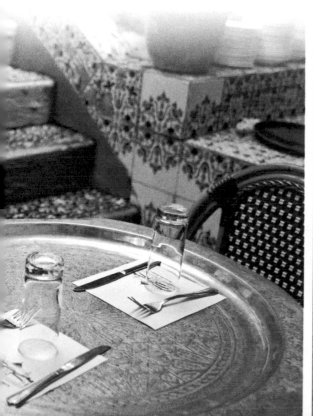

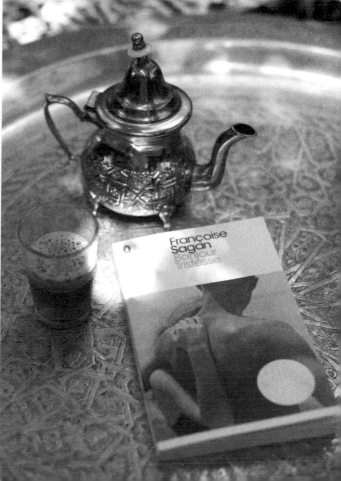

MOROCCAN MINT TEA

My obsession with Moroccan mint tea began on a romantic date at Le 404 in the Upper Marais. After our tasty tagines and couscous, our waiter served the sweet minty hot tea, and to my delight, I was hooked, and so was my cute date. So much so that the following afternoon we made our way to the Latin Quarter for more at the Grand Mosque. Here we entered another world I'd had no idea existed in Paris: a serene haven of teal-colored tile mosaics, a shaded cozy café, a Moroccan restaurant, and an array of Middle Eastern pastries.

We chose a table in the garden café surrounded by Parisians and some tiny birds swimming in a fountain. Some tables were filled with groups of girlfriends; some guests were, like me, on a date; and a few Latin Quarter girls were alone, sipping mint tea and reading French novels. What a perfect neighborhood spot to relax and read a book in a tranquil space while enjoying tea and non-French pastry.

I love to make the tea when I'm home alone or to enjoy with my boyfriend. It's a fun reminder of the one of many times I dragged him to Paris with me.

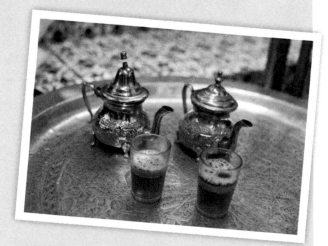

Moroccan Mint Tea

- 2 tablespoons Chinese gunpowder tea or green tea
- 16 lumps sugar or 1/3 cup granulated sugar
- 1 bunch mint, stems discarded (about 25 sprigs)

Place tea, sugar, mint, and 4 cups boiling water in a teapot and stir until sugar dissolves; let sit for 10 minutes.

To serve, strain tea into serving glasses.

Serves 4 to 6

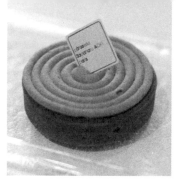

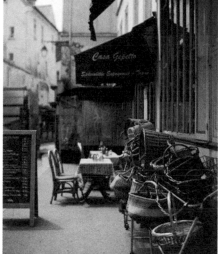

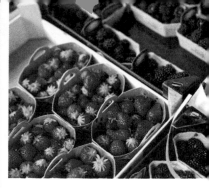

Sadaharu Aoki
56, Boulevard de Port Royal

At this sweet spot, a Japanese pastry chef creates unique treats, mixing Japanese ingredients with classic French-style pastries. It's a bit out of the way, but it's a true pleasure to sit with a cup of Japanese tea and enjoy the most delicious salty caramel tarte.

Maison Claudel Vin et Whisky
62, Rue Monge

This wine and whisky bar is a favorite neighborhood date spot of the Latin Quarter girl. She enjoys a wine tasting while her beau sips a whisky flight and together they enjoy a cheese-and-charcuterie platter.

La Maison des Trois Thés
1, Rue Saint Médard

Tea lovers and connoisseurs stop into this off-the-beaten-path tea salon for a very special experience: to learn tea rituals from Madame Yu Hui Tseng, the only female master of the Chinese Tea Ceremony in the world. Madame Tseng serves more than a thousand blends of Chinese tea, some even dating back to the early 1900s.

Rue Mouffetard

One of Paris's oldest medieval streets is home to a lively fresh vegetable and fruit market, gourmet food shops, and cafés. Walking down this pedestrian cobblestone street, you will encounter Latin Quarter women of all ages. It's fun to people watch as they shop for fresh fruit, visit the fish market, and sample the wares at the cheese shop.

Le Verre à Pied
118, Bis Rue Mouffetard

A bar and *tabac* buzzing with locals throughout the day and live music a few nights a week. Catch a glimpse of old-fashioned Paris, as its décor has not changed much since the early 1900s. If you can't make it to Paris, watch the film *Amélie* and see the bar in the scene where she eavesdrops on Mr. Bretodeau sharing his delight in finding his box of keepsakes.

Le Boulangerie de Monge
123, Rue Monge

One of the best boulangeries (bread shops) in Paris, with a line out the door on weekends. Take a peek through the window as they make the breads on-site. As you leave, do as the Parisians do and take a bite out of the end of the crust to enjoy your fresh warm baguette right away.

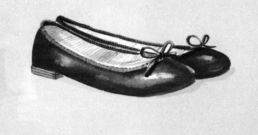

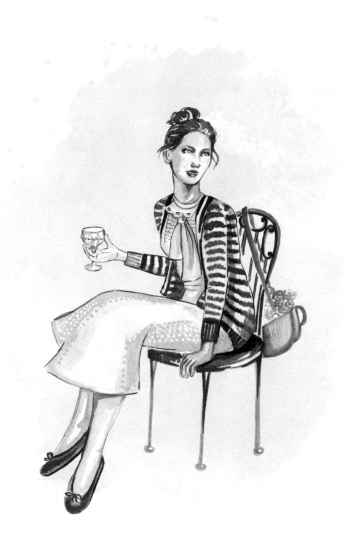

CHAPTER 11
SAINT-GERMAIN

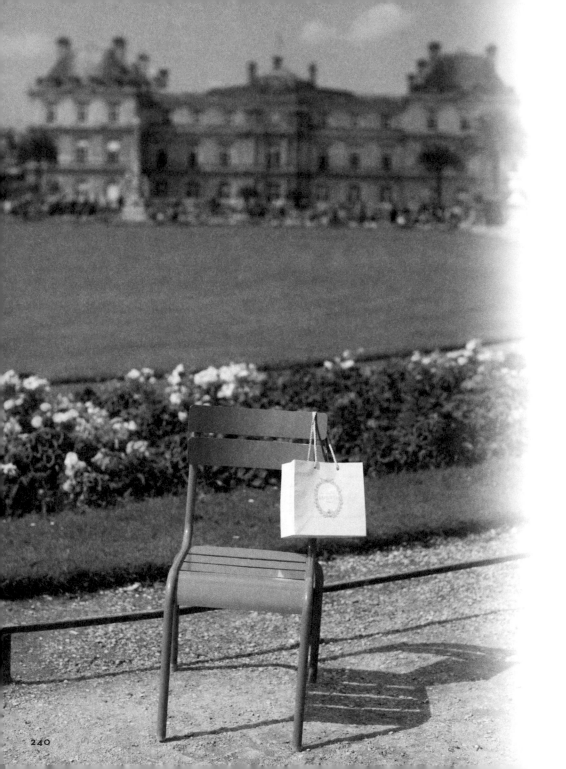

Waking up in Saint-Germain, you'll notice something special in the air. Your day may begin with a usual routine, but once you step outside it will be anything but ordinary. In Saint-Germain, the ladies aren't just walking along the boulevards; they float. One by one, they exit their apartments, elegant and chic, floating along to work at one of the area's many antique shops and art galleries. With hair up in a bun and a uniform of A-line skirt, ballet flats, and striped Sonia Rykiel cardigan, the Saint-Germain woman is the most classically chic Parisian woman in the most classically chic Parisian neighborhood.

Saint-Germain is an amazing mix of city and village. One minute you're walking along the bustling boulevard Saint-Germain with designer boutiques and packed cafés, and the next you find yourself wandering down rue de Verneuil, so peaceful and charming you'll feel like you've gone back in time one hundred years. The neighborhood boasts Paris's oldest department store, Le Bon Marché, with an amazing mix of contemporary and designer collections, a nail bar, and an epic gourmet food store. When you've shopped till you drop, head to the tranquil Luxembourg Gardens. You'll find they're full of life—young and old—with fountains, sculptures, and petite Parisian-girls-in-training playing games with their friends.

Like her low-profile arrondissement, the Saint-Germain woman is charming but discreet. She enjoys hosting dinner parties at home and meeting girlfriends at Les Deux Magots for a glass of rosé, and, like Karl Lagerfeld, she is a late-night regular at Café des Flore. She shops for timeless items in her wardrobe that can translate each season and year after year in a palette of distinctive grays, blacks, and neutrals with just a touch of color. Splurges on made-to-order accessories that she will never outgrow complete her never-overdressed-yet-never-underdressed approach to dressing. An antique expert, when shopping for her home, she regularly visits Paris's best flea markets in search of classic yet unique pieces.

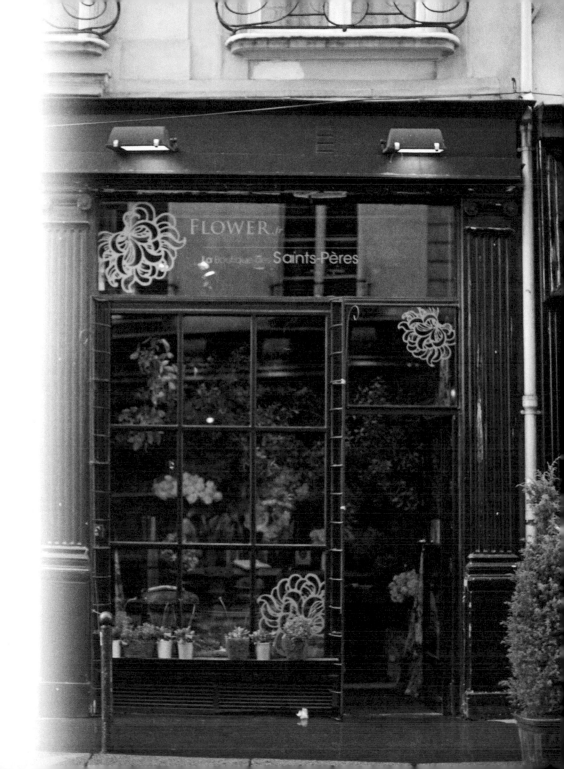

La Palette
43, Rue de Seine

A Parisian bobo hangout on a quiet corner in Saint-Germain, here you'll find a laid-back bohemian vibe, great wine, and artists' paint palettes that date back as far as the 1920s hanging on the walls. Heaters keep the outdoor terrace vibrant even during the winter months.

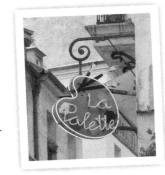

Bar du Marché
75, Rue de Seine

Their signature red-and-white striped awning welcomes Parisians to this fun pedestrian street full of cafés and bars. By far the standout spot on the block, this bar is one of my favorite meeting points to start a night with drinks and a tasty side of French fries before dinner.

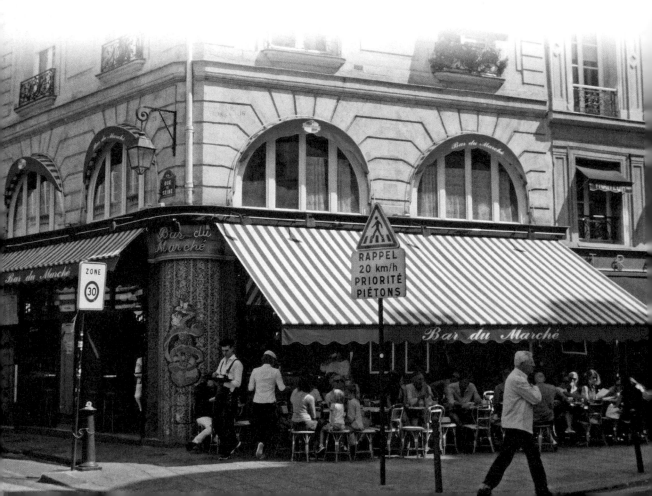

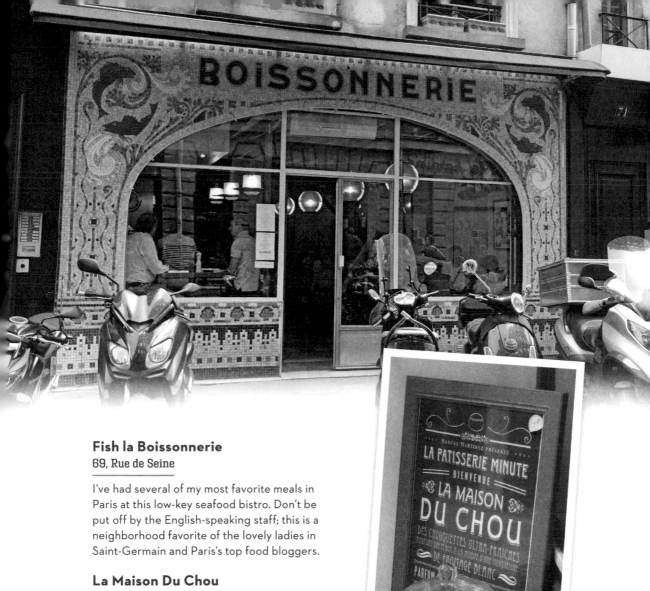

Fish la Boissonnerie
69, Rue de Seine

I've had several of my most favorite meals in
Paris at this low-key seafood bistro. Don't be
put off by the English-speaking staff; this is a
neighborhood favorite of the lovely ladies in
Saint-Germain and Paris's top food bloggers.

La Maison Du Chou
7, Rue de Furstenberg

Tucked away on a tiny tree-lined square is a
hidden gem that I'm sure Parisians would
prefer to keep hidden. Fresh cream puffs are
filled to order with a variety of flavor options.
If you're in the need to cure a tiny sweet tooth,
you can pick up just one... or three.

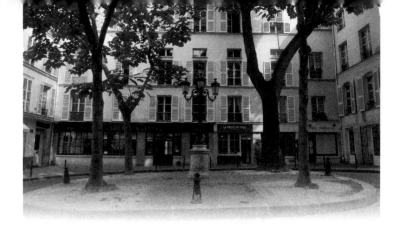

Prescription Cocktail Club
23, Rue Mazarine

This is a favorite cocktail bar for the ladies of Saint-Germain. Perfect whether they are meeting friends or on a date, it is large enough to not feel too cramped but still has a very intimate vibe. The signature cocktail, Rouge George, is infused with an exotic mix of Rittenhouse whisky, Santa Teresa rum, vermouth, and a dash of orange zest.

Musée National Eugène Delacroix
6, Rue de Furstenberg

The museum's garden is a secret spot for Saint-Germain girls to spend a few quiet hours of reading on a Sunday afternoon. The former apartment and studio of the Romantic painter showcases his paintings, sketches, and drawings.

THE JAZZ AGE

Step into the 1950s jazz era of Paris. The ladies of Saint-Germain are entertained with live jazz music almost every night of the week. A few of their neighborhood haunts . . .

CAFÉ LAURENT, 33, Rue Dauphine
For date night with her man, the Saint-Germain girl can sit in the jazz room here or enjoy a cozy conversation by the fireplace in the lounge with jazz playing in the background.

PARIS-PRAGUE JAZZ CLUB, 18, Rue Bonaparte
Hidden in an ancient stone cellar at the Czech center, they showcase jazz musicians from all over the world.

CHEZ PAPA, 3, Rue Saint-Benoît
Intimate jazz setting with delicious food Tuesday through Saturday nights. Photos of past performers hanging on the walls, from as far back as the 1950s, bring you back in time.

Ladurée
21, Rue Bonaparte

At one of the most beautiful locations of the famous pâtisserie and salon de thé, the jewel-toned mural of exotic peacocks in a secret garden and light streaming through the canopy ceiling transports you to a magical land.

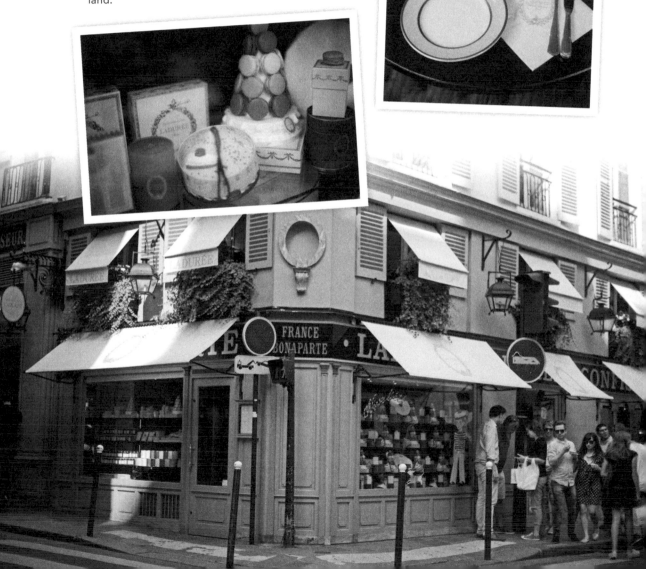

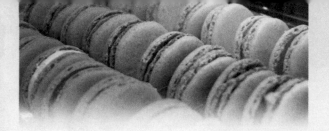

THE FRENCH MACARON CHALLENGE

Currently, one of the most talked about food competitions is definitely Ladurée vs. Pierre Hermé macarons. Remember the Coke versus Pepsi taste challenge in the 1980s? Yes, this is just as serious. First, let's start with the basics. A macaron is two meringue discs with a creamy flavored ganache center. It's a delicious bite that's flakey and gooey all at once. It's tough to master, but Ladurée and Pierre Hermé have done just that. They make them to perfection every time.

Ladurée has more classic flavors, like raspberry, vanilla, and chocolate, while Pierre Hermé flavors walk a bit on the wild side: olive oil with mandarin, chocolate and foie gras—you get the idea. His imaginative and exotic flavor combinations hit the mark. Some think Pierre Hermé uses too much ganache and thus the macaron is too gooey, while others like that most about his macarons. Although simpler, the flavors of Laudrée macarons are outstanding and bold, and the meringue is light as air. People pass through the doors at Ladurée not just for the macarons, but for the experience of sitting in their pastel-colored tea salon. It's quite dreamy, and when it's filled with the girls of Saint-Germain, you may feel like you're dining among princesses.

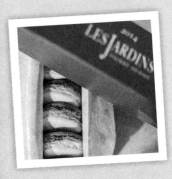

Both pâtisseries have locations on the same street, just a few blocks apart in Saint-Germain. So when you're in Paris, mingle in line with the ladies of this arrondissement and take the challenge for yourself. Then try making your own at home. Be patient—it usually takes a few tries to bake the meringue without it cracking.

Lauderée, 21, Rue Bonaparte

Pierre Hermé, 72, Rue Bonaparte

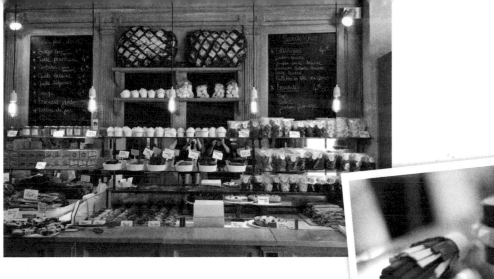

Joséphine Bakery
42, Rue Jacob

The décor here is as chic as the Saint-Germain ladies who frequent this bakery. You'll spot them picking up coffee and a breakfast treat on the way to work or stopping in for lunch before heading back to work.

Huilerie Artisanale J. Leblanc et Fils
12, Rue Jacob

For four generations, the Leblanc family has ground and pressed high-quality seeds and nuts to produce some of the finest cooking oils, vinegars, and mustards in France. Their staff at the boutique can help make suggestions as to which oils to pair with your cooking and even arrange a tour of their factory in southern Burgundy. I love using the pumpkin oil and pistachio oil not just for cooking; both are equally delicious as salad dressings.

Ragtime
23, Rue de l'Echaudé

You can get lost for hours in this vintage boutique. Daydream about the ladies who wore the pristine gowns from the 1930s and the life they experienced while wearing them.

Gab & Jo
28, Rue Jacob

This Parisian concept shop has an eclectic mix of accessories, objets d'art, and home décor items. Everything is unique, stylish, and made by up-and-coming French brands and artisans, some exclusive to the boutique. Strike up a conversation with the enthusiastic shop owner, who will be happy to share the backstory behind brands and merchandise he hand selects.

L'Hotel
13, Rue des Beaux Arts

This magical hotel in Saint-Germain is filled with great moments in history. Oscar Wilde lived and died on its magnificent steps. Princess Grace, Salvador Dalí, Frank Sinatra, and Elizabeth Taylor have all lived here for periods of time. The Saint-Germain girl loves its understated glamour and stops by regularly for some of the best cocktails in town.

La Crèmerie
9, Rue des Quatre Vents

Located in a former late-nineteenth-century dairy shop, this wine bar and store is tucked away on a quiet street. It serves organic natural wines with fresh charcuterie from artisanal producers in France, Italy, and Spain.

Binome
5, Rue de Condé

Two friends both named Delphine opened this boutique. One designs super-cool jewelry, the other leather totes and shoes. You will find their designs mixed in with other under-the-radar collections.

L'Avant Comptoir
9, Carrefour de l'Odeon

Parisians don't mind a wine bar that's standing-room only when the food is by Chef Yves Camdeborde. Try the skewer of seared foie gras with roasted red peppers and Iberian ham croquettes.

Marie-Hélène de Taillac
8, Rue de Tournon

This fine jewelry designer uses delicate, colorful jewels to create the most beautiful statement pieces. Lipstick-red couch, blue walls, and chandeliers that look like giant pearls give the shop a chic and modern feel.

Huîtrerié Regis
3, Rue de Montfaucon

A tiny oyster bar on a tiny street. The cute white décor and cottage feel will transport you to the coast of Brittany.

Compagnie des Vins Surnaturels
7, Rue Lobineau

This wine bar from the Paris cocktail experts at Experimental and Prescription offers a wide selection at a wide range of prices. Serving wine by the glass, bottle, or pitcher, they also have plates of ham, truffles, and cheese that will delight your taste buds.

Les Trois Marches de Catherine B
1, Rue Guisarde

One of the few places in the world you can find yourself surrounded by a room full of vintage Chanel and Hermés bags, this shop also houses an impressive collection of vintage Hermés silk scarves and Chanel costume jewelry. Catherine's boutique next door, selling clothing and vintage shoes, is by appointment only.

Attal Nessim
122, Rue d'Assas

Come here to purchase custom-made shoes. You get to pick the leather, color, and style—from open-toe T-straps to gladiator sandals with a wedge heel. Expect a waiting list for your shoes, as almost all Saint-Germain girls and Parisian fashion editors order their summer sandals from Nessim.

A HEAVENLY SCENTED HOME

Like the importance of a signature fragrance, French women feel that a signature scent for their home is also vital. And no better way to scent your home than with candles. The French have brought luxury and craftsmanship back into the art of candle making.

Almost as important as the scent is the look and design. Parisian women want to match their candles to their home décor, and not just any candle will do. That's where Cire Trudon—a candle maker since the seventeenth century—comes in, bringing specialty scents to candle lovers everywhere.

Manufacturing their candles in the same workshop in Normandy that supplied candles to the court of King Louis XIV, Cire Trudon bases its work on three standards: know-how, perfume, and history.

Master candle makers for hundreds of years, they carry on the tradition of fine craftsmanship and superior materials. Their candles, available in twenty-four dreamy scents and three sizes, are housed in a green glass that is handmade in Italy in the shape of a champagne bucket. The glass is adorned with a gold label that includes the coat of arms of King Louis XIV, a beehive, and the Cire Trudon motto, which translates to: "Bees work for God and for the king."

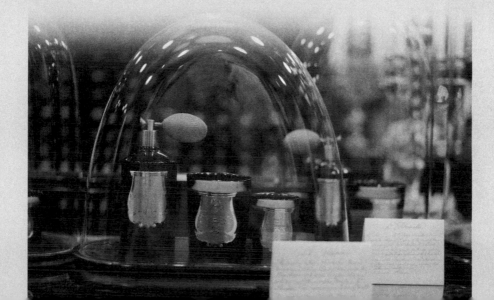

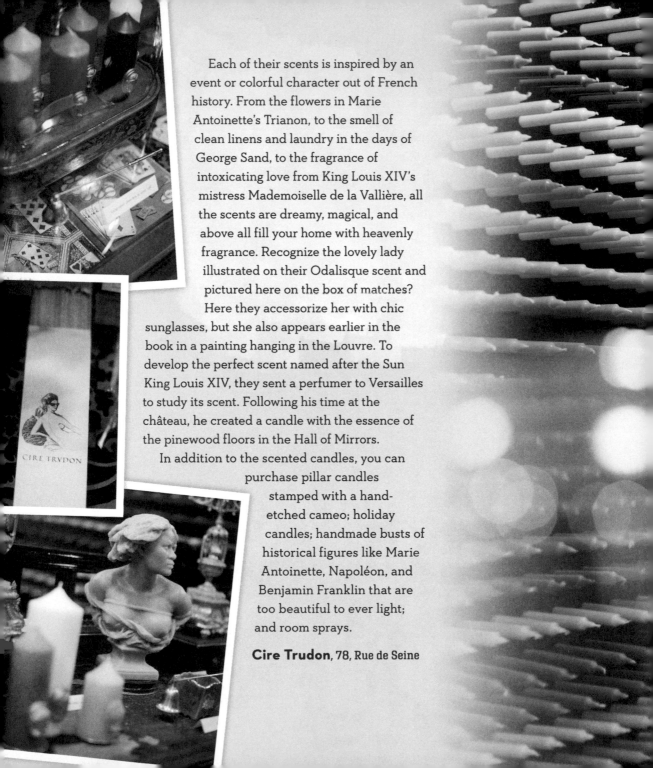

Each of their scents is inspired by an event or colorful character out of French history. From the flowers in Marie Antoinette's Trianon, to the smell of clean linens and laundry in the days of George Sand, to the fragrance of intoxicating love from King Louis XIV's mistress Mademoiselle de la Vallière, all the scents are dreamy, magical, and above all fill your home with heavenly fragrance. Recognize the lovely lady illustrated on their Odalisque scent and pictured here on the box of matches? Here they accessorize her with chic sunglasses, but she also appears earlier in the book in a painting hanging in the Louvre. To develop the perfect scent named after the Sun King Louis XIV, they sent a perfumer to Versailles to study its scent. Following his time at the château, he created a candle with the essence of the pinewood floors in the Hall of Mirrors.

In addition to the scented candles, you can purchase pillar candles stamped with a hand-etched cameo; holiday candles; handmade busts of historical figures like Marie Antoinette, Napoléon, and Benjamin Franklin that are too beautiful to ever light; and room sprays.

Cire Trudon, 78, Rue de Seine

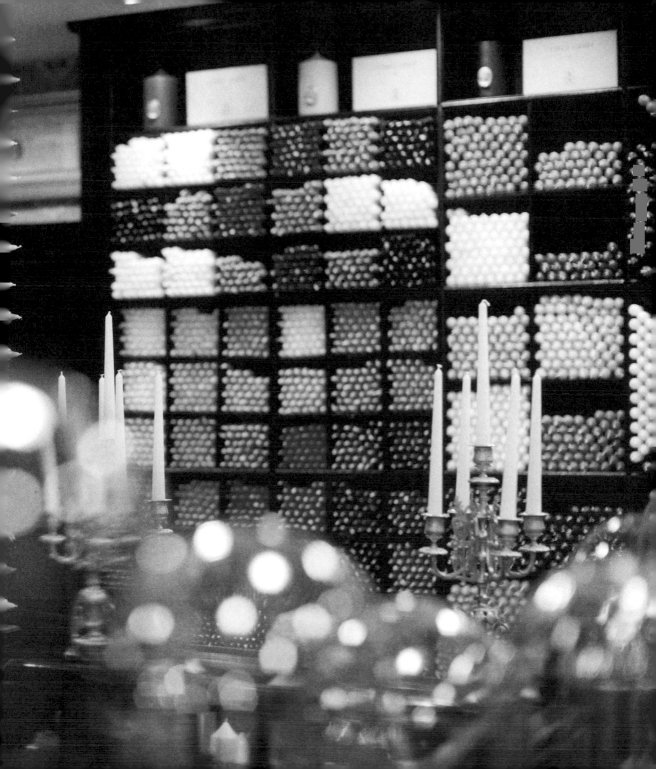

Jardin du Luxembourg
Rue de Vaugirard and Rue de Medicis

This beautiful park spans sixty acres, with
more than one hundred statues, fountains,
and monuments. Musée du Luxembourg
hosts temporary art exhibits, while the
terraces hold statues of France's queens
and female saints. Once you've explored
the gardens, take a seat in one of the
mint-green reclining chairs and take
notice of the Saint-Germain ladies
wandering through or catching up with
their girlfriends. Study their style long
enough and you can pinpoint which
neighborhood each lives in.

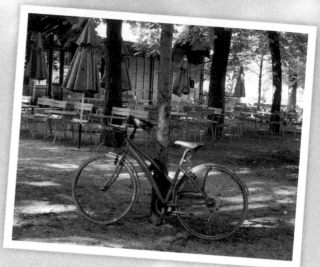

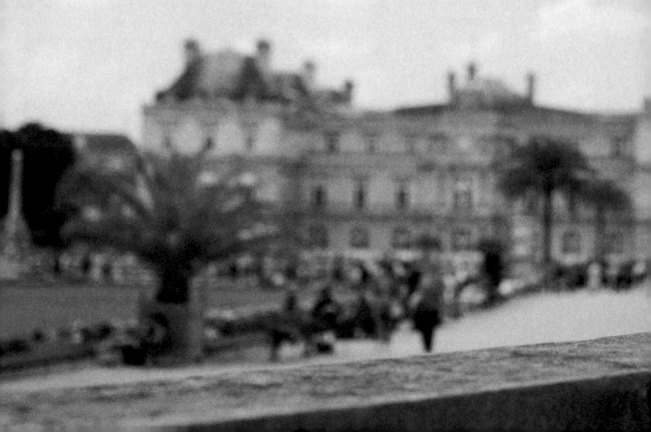

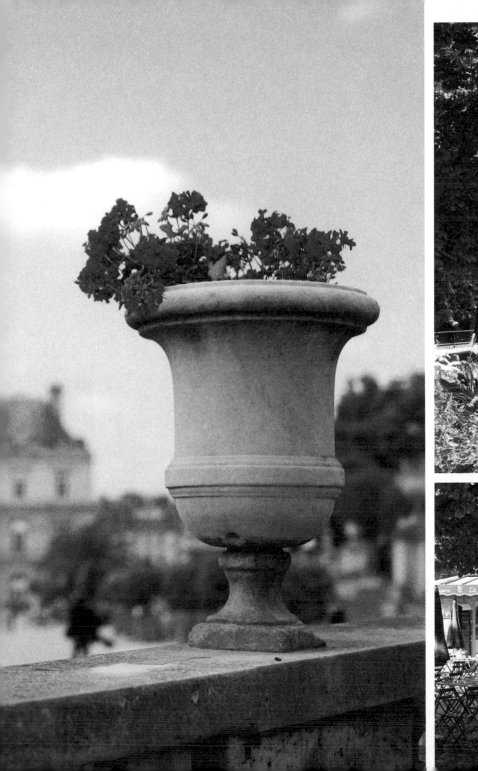
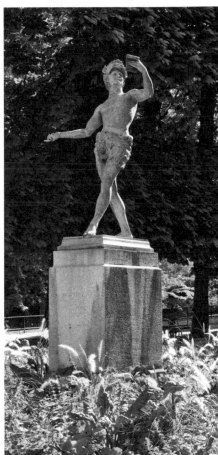
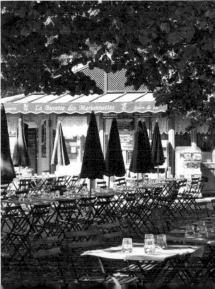

13-A Baker's Dozen
16, Rue des Saints-Pères

At the end of a tiny cobblestone courtyard you'll find this charming café, and as soon as you enter you'll feel right at home. Mixing southern family recipes and charm with the freshest French produce and spices, owner, chef, and baker Laurel Sanderson creates the golden ticket for a delicious breakfast or lunch. Pick up a copy of one of my favorite cookbooks, David Lebovitz's, *My Paris Kitchen*, which includes the recipe for Laurel's mouthwatering carrot cake.

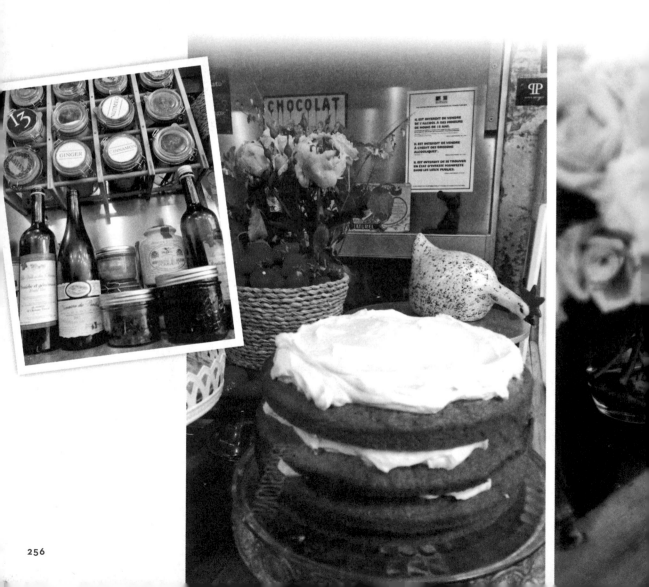

La Boutique des Saints-Pères
14, Rue des Saints-Pères

Step into this flower shop and into *A Midsummer Night's Dream*. I can't walk through Saint-Germain without stopping in and saying hello to the floral artists who create the most beautiful arrangements. Thank heavens for Instagram, where I can still see their new creations even when I'm not in Paris.

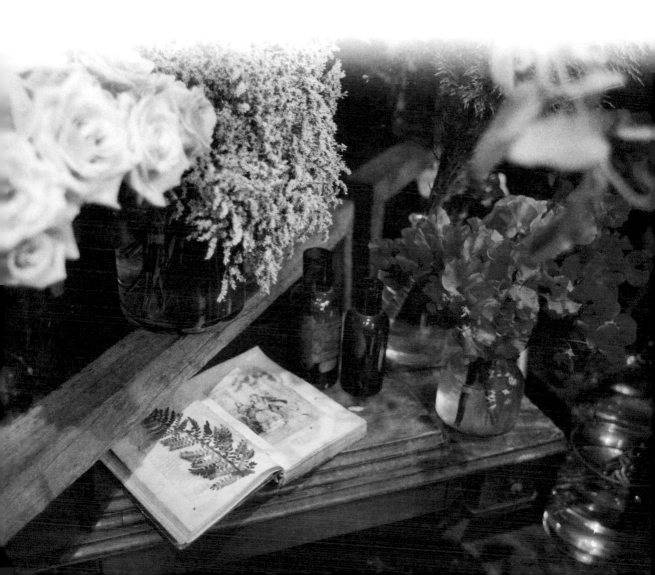

–Blake Lively, ACTRESS AND FOUNDER OF PRESERVE.US

Paris is a city that serves the senses. For my eyes, I never get tired of gawking at Monet's *Water Lilies* at Musée de l'Orangerie. For my taste buds, oh boy, nothing is kinder to them than a feast by Jean-François Piège. For my ears, I find goofy, childlike joy in the sounds of the music boxes at puppet shop Claire de Rêve. For my nose, I drink in the scents filling the magical canisters at Mariage Frères. For the pleasure of touch, stops on rue Saint-Honorè at Fifi Chachnil and Chantal Thomass are a necessary guilty pleasure. And for my feet (yes, they count as a sense while in Paris), a visit to the atelier of the enchanting Christian Louboutin reminds a girl that she's never too old to pretend she's Cinderella.

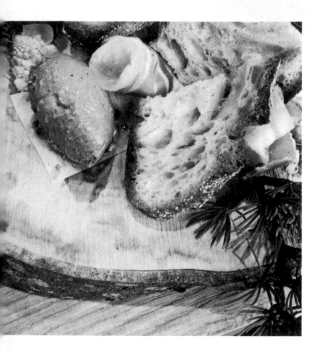

Clover
5, Rue Perronet

Chef Jean-François Piège and wife, Elodie, recently opened this intimate *restaurant du quartier*, which shows as much heart in its food as they do for each other. The freshest ingredients are sourced to create witty dishes like Piège's scallops served on a Parisian cobblestone and Armoise Chicken served with a strip of incredible Comté rice cake inspired by a recipe of his grandmother's. This instant neighborhood favorite seats just twenty diners, so better make your reservations far in advance.

Comtesse du Barry
1, Rue de Sèvres

Foie Gras, terrines, truffles, caviar, and just about any other decadent food item you can think of can be found at this boutique named after the last chief mistress of King Louis XV. The rainbow of terrines on display is to foodies what a wall of paint colors at Home Depot is to a painter. . . . Pure delight.

CAFÉ CULTURE

Café culture is quintessentially French, and there's no better place to learn about this aspect of French life than in Saint-Germain, with its wonderful selection of cafés. Throughout history, Parisians have treated the Paris café as an extension of their apartments. It's the place to work, read, and catch up with friends. So when in Saint-Germain, spend time at Café de Flore like Simone de Beauvoir or next door on the terrace at Les Deux Magots. Don't forget your dark sunglasses, which are a must-have accessory for discreet people watching and studying the Saint-Germain woman in her natural habitat.

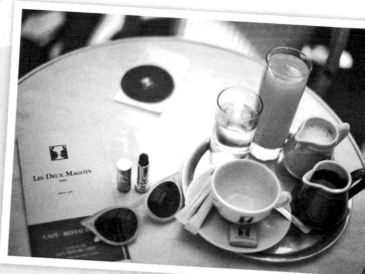

LES DEUX MAGOTS, 6, Place Saint-Germain-des-Prés
For a perfectly Parisian relaxing afternoon, choose a table located on the side terrace and a bottle of rosé wine.

CAFÉ DE FLORE, 172, Boulevard Saint-Germain
The most fashionable spot in all of Paris. If you're lucky to see an empty table outside, grab it. Or head to the upstairs dining room for a bite. Whether for coffee at 10 a.m. or a midnight croque monsieur, you will be in the midst of the chicest Parisians of all ages.

Brasserie Lipp
151, Boulevard Saint-Germain

One of my favorite brasseries in Paris, it has been serving classic French dishes since 1870 to a who's who in art, film, politics, and the literary world. Imagine sitting at a table across from Hemingway, Proust, or Gregory Peck. After you've finished dinner, hop across the street to get a nightcap at Café de Flores for a full Parisian experience.

Eggs & Co
11, Rue Bernard Palissy

Serving eggs all day, seven days a week, they offer your choice of fluffy omelettes or perfecly poached, scrambled, or fried eggs, with many meat and veggie options mixed in or on the side. It's a small café, so with brunch this delicious, you need a reservation on the weekends.

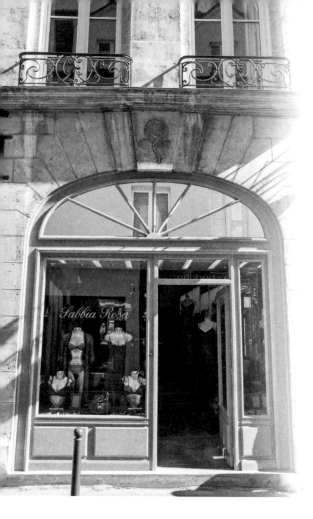

Poilâne
8, Rue du Cherche Midi

One of the most famous boulangeries in the world, their signature item is the round sourdough loaf stamped with a P. Saint-Germain women will stop by on their way to a picnic in nearby Luxembourg Gardens. If you're craving this baker's bread from home, they happily ship worldwide and you can receive a fresh loaf within forty-eight hours of the order.

La Cuisine de Bar/Poilâne
8, Rue du Cherche-Midi

A petite lunch spot that specializes in toasted open-faced sandwiches on the famous Poilâne pain de champagne country bread. Stamped with a signature P, the loaf is made with just four ingredients—sourdough, stone-ground wheat flour, water, and sea salt, and cooked to crunchy perfection in a wood-burning oven. Enjoy your tartine with smoked salmon and crème fraîche, tomato and melted mozzarella, and many other delectable combinations for breakfast and lunch.

Gertrude Stein's Residence
27, Rue de Fleurus

The great American writer and art collector who was brought to life by Kathy Bates in *Midnight in Paris* lived at this address and hosted the great literary and art world in the 1920s. That's a home and era I'd love to travel back in time to experience.

Sabbia Rosa
73, Rue Des Saints-Pères

A small boudoir-style lingerie shop with incredible pieces worth every euro. Once you're in the fitting room, they will take your measurements and then bring you bra options that they feel are best for your body type and in colors that look best on your skin color. These Parisian women know a thing or two about bras and never go wrong.

Repetto
51, Rue du Four

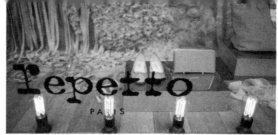

The company used to only design ballet slippers for the world's prima ballerinas, but when Brigitte Bardot requested a ballerina slipper to wear throughout the day, Rose Repetto happily obliged, and the rest is history. This is not just a Saint-Germain girls' staple; all Parisian girls have at least one pair, available to them in a rainbow of colors.

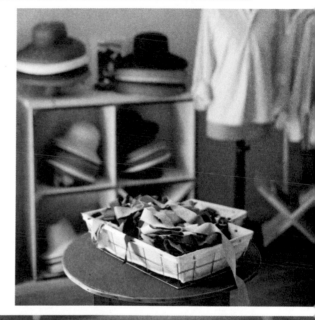

La Cerise sur le Chapeau
11, Rue Cassette

A cute hat boutique where you get to be the designer. Saint-Germain women love to create their own wardrobe pieces, and here they can select from styles inspired by different eras. Select your style, fabric, and color trims, and the talented ladies at the boutique will create your chapeau, usually finished in the same day. Enjoy some tea at the hotel across the street while you wait.

Jean-Charles Rochoux
16, Rue d'Assas

An incredible chocolatier that's a hidden gem among the chain chocolate shops in Paris, Rochoux's enchanting chocolate animals and sculptured busts of famous emperors look almost too perfect to eat. One item I never leave without is the hazelnut-and-forest-strawberry spread.

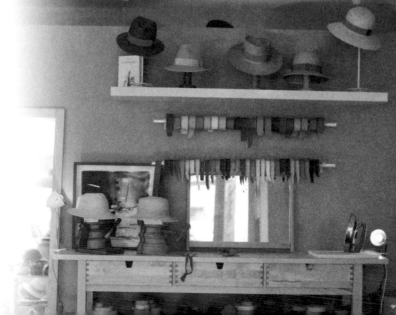

GET THE
SAINT-GERMAIN LOOK

Ballet Flats

So simple and chic they go with just about anything, except perhaps a red-carpet gown. You can buy these just about anywhere. After my ultimate favorite flats, Repetto, chic and affordable styles by Yosi Samra are my next go-to. I still dream of having my very own Chanel flats, which I've heard from Parisian girlfriends are extremely comfortable.

Cardigan

I live in cardigans year-round. They are the perfect layering piece, whether over a summer dress or a T-shirt, or as an extra layer on a cold winter's day. Cardigan sweaters don't have to be simple. Saint-Germain girls wear solid-colored cashmere, and they also love Sonia Rykiel's assortment of bold stripes and bright colors. They add a little bit of quirky to this girl's chic look.

Trench Coat

The trench coat is a wardrobe staple for most women around the globe. Either belted or unbelted, the trench looks chic over just about everything from jeans and cigarette pants to dresses. Find the perfect avant-garde styles by Lahssan, or go for classic looks by Coach, which has mastered the trench in crisp cottons, soft leather, and lightweight wool.

Maison Jules

Knowing the love American girls have for French style, Macy's recently launched an exclusive collection inspired by our favorite Parisian staples. Maison Jules is full of all our French style favorites, from striped boatneck tops to flirty dresses, knit cardigans, and chic sweaters. All at affordable prices. One of my favorite Parisian insiders, Betty Autier, is the perfect choice as a brand ambassador.

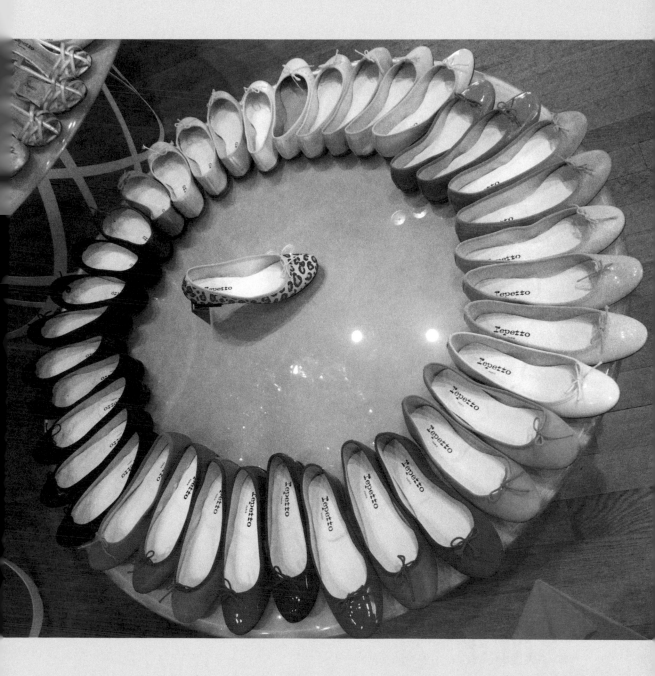

Le Bon Marché
24, Rue de Sèvres

Paris's first department store, with contemporary designer and luxury collections for men and women and an amazing gourmet food department. This is where Parisians go to create a look with a mix of Parisian must-haves from Sandro, Helmut Lang, Petit Bateau, and Adieu loafers. Le Théâtre de la Beauté carries selections from the best fragrance houses under one roof and includes a modern nail bar which offers a quick polish change for under 10 euro. If you need a shopping break, join the Saint-Germain girl at Délicabar for lunch.

La Grande Épicerie de Paris is a beautiful space with more than three thousand gourmet products from around the globe. It's a food lover's dream, with case upon case of pastries, fresh fish, meat, and pasta; shelves of exotic spices, mustards, and jams; and a wine and champagne department.

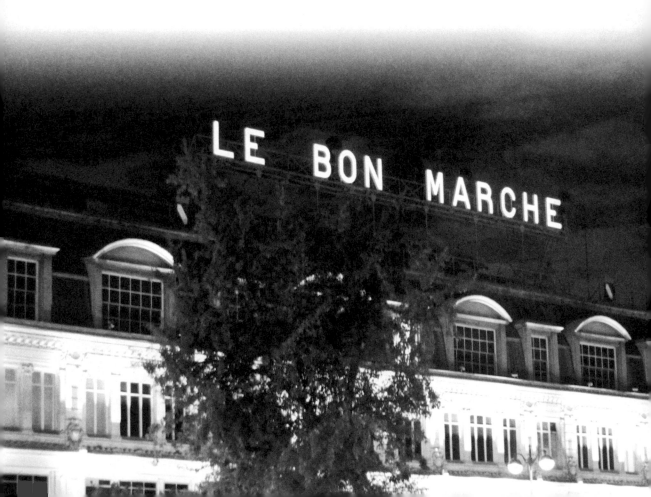

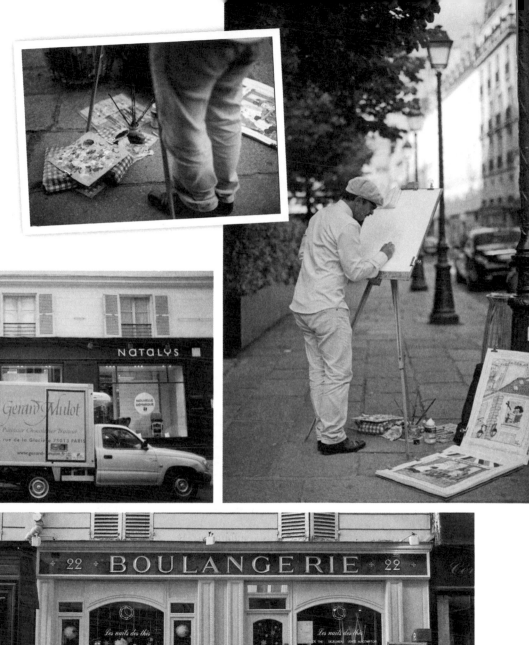
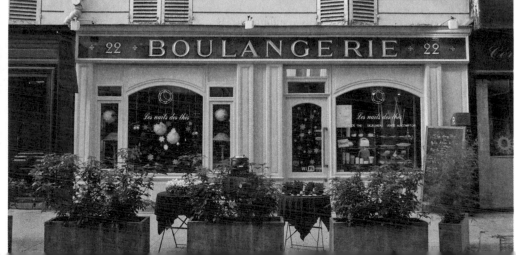

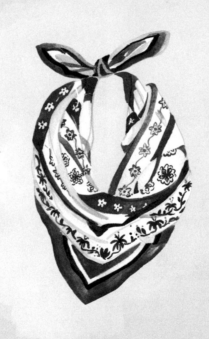

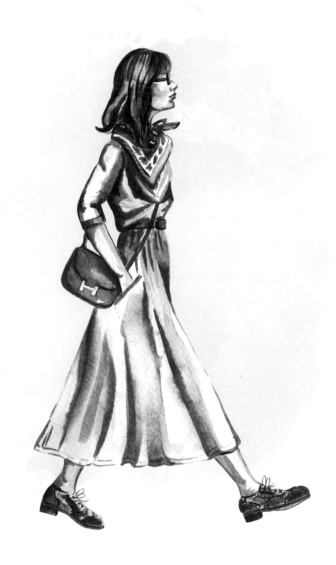

CHAPTER 12
CHAMP DE MARS

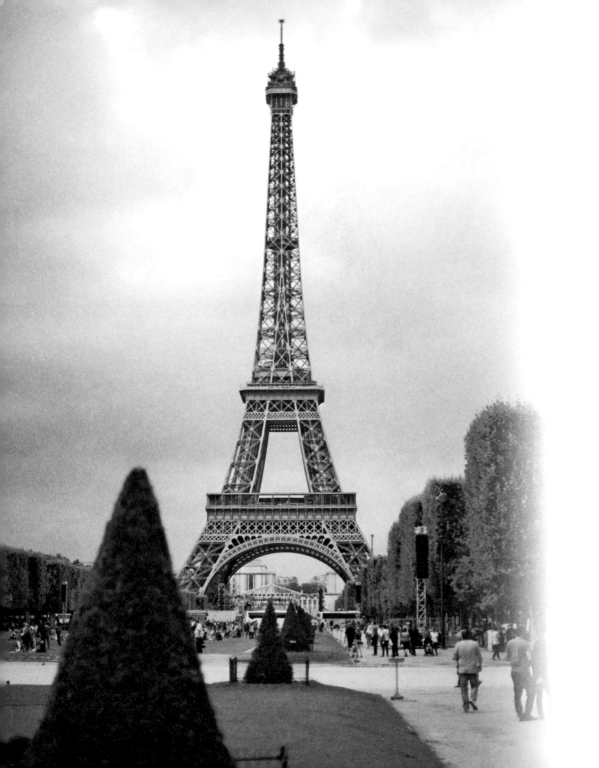

Residing in the arrondissement still associated with French nobility, the Champ de Mars woman is a true classic—but by no means boring. She's casual chic in Oxford flats and a flowy skirt, with a printed silk scarf in muted tones to pull together her look without overpowering it. She shops for French classics at Comptoir de Cotonniers and Petit Bateau, and heads to Claude Pierlot for a more dressed-up look to wear on a date night with her husband.

A young, stylish mom, after she drops her kids at school, she begins her day reading *Le Figaro* at Coutume Café, and on occasion will meet up with girlfriends for lunch at Les Cocottes. She and her family spend free time strolling the sculpture garden at Musée Rodin. They prefer to join their neighbors for a picnic at Place des Invalides and leave Jardin du Champ de Mars, next to the Eiffel Tower, for the tourists to picnic. On the way over, they pick up the world's best sliced ham at Bellota-Bellota and cheese from one of the many award-winning fromageries that are all close by.

The Champ de Mars woman enjoys a peaceful afternoon at the tranquil tea garden at the La Pagode movie theater. A Japanese hidden oasis in the heart of Paris, it was the setting for an infamous Parisian scandal. Befriend a local Parisian woman and maybe she will open up about this Parisian secret. There's never a dull moment even in the most conservative of neighborhoods in Paris.

With more open markets than any other area in Paris, the Champ de Mars woman has her choice, any day of the week. On weekends she tends to shop on the cobblestone rue Cler, with fresh food shops and cafés that stay busy throughout the day. On Sundays, she prefers rue de Grenelle's market, which includes an antique section in the morning.

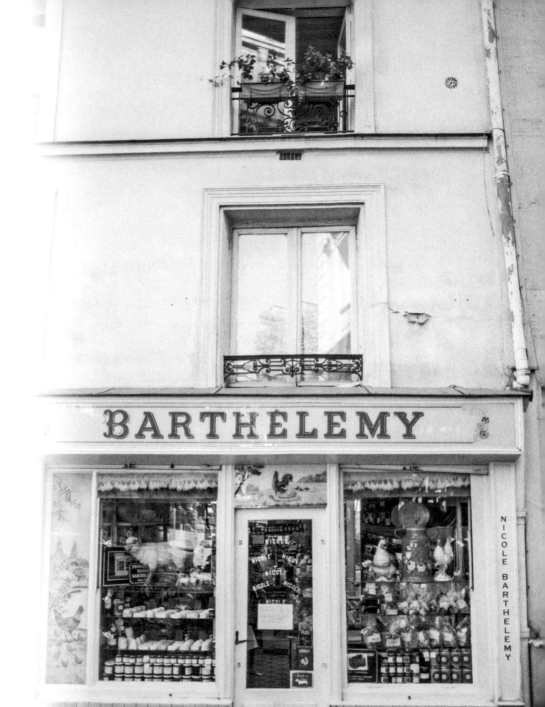

WRAP YOURSELF
THE PARISIAN WAY

We've all read about this style phenomenon, seen it depicted in film and television, and I'm sure have had at least one conversation with our girlfriends about the topic: French women and their scarves. Even more of an iconic French style, I think, than a Chanel bag or Louboutins, a scarf is an accessory French women of all ages, styles, and budgets wear year-round. This was most definitely a French-girl experience I needed to learn for myself.

One of my favorite scenes in the film *Le Divorce* starring Kate Hudson, Naomi Watts, and Glenn Close, was when Glenn Close so perfectly describes to Kate Hudson some of the many different ways French women wear their scarves—

"Knotted in front, one end down and the other end thrown over the shoulder, or looped around and doubled with the ends tucked in, or around the shoulder over the coat like a shawl, or tied in the back." And then she went on to list different words the French have for "scarf."

Her description of what to many women is more a functional accessory than a fashionable one is so delightful, I wanted to run to my scarf drawer and immediately throw one on. When in Paris, it's such a treat to walk down a boulevard and see Parisian women wear their scarves all of the different ways.

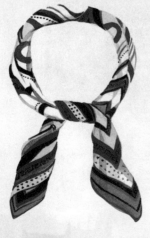 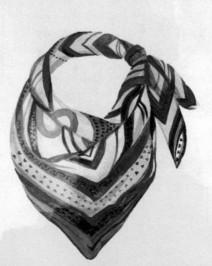 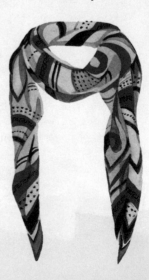

—Georgina Chapman and Keren Craig, COFOUNDERS OF MARCHESA

I love that Paris will always be Paris. Its beauty remains unchanged and the magic always works. Whenever we're in Paris we always go to Deyrolle, famed for taxidermy since the early nineteenth century. Their collection and cabinets of curiosity are peerless. A few doors up, do not forget to sample La Pâtisserie des Rêves's Paris-Brest.

Simone
1, Rue de Saint-Simon

Champ de Mars ladies stop in here to see the latest from contemporary designers, both established and up-and-coming. They find dresses from one of their favorite U.K. designers, Orla Kiely, and Antik Batik accessories perfect for an upcoming vacation in Morocco.

Deyrolle
46, Rue du Bac

Remember the Montmartre wedding scene in *Midnight in Paris*? It was shot in this witty taxidermy and curiosity shop. Stop by to see the collection of butterflies, insects, microscopic instruments, and rare curiosities.

Chocolat Chapon
69, Rue du Bac

The former official ice-cream maker for Buckingham Palace has returned home to France and opened this award-winning pâtisserie. When you can indulge in truffles, chocolates, ice cream, and smoked salted pralines, what more do you need? Chapon has decided it's a chocolate mousse bar....

La Pâtisserie des Rêves
93, Rue du Bac

The pastries are just as delicious as they are beautiful at this pâtisserie famous for baking the best Paris-Brest in its namesake city.

Epicerie Générale
43, Rue de Verneuil

An adorable French general store selling organic fresh fruits, vegetables, gourmet jelly, and a small selection of meats and cheeses from local producers and farms.

Musée d'Orsay
1, Rue de la Legion d'Honneur

This impressionist art museum is filled with inspiring artwork by Monet, Van Gogh, Renoir, and more. Built during Le Belle Epoque, it was the first train station in Paris, and it is a regular place to find the Saint-Germain girls wandering through for inspiration. Their café on the top floor has amazing views of the Sacré-Cœur in Montmartre.

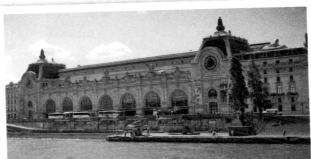

L'Arpege
84, Rue de Varenne

With a menu almost exclusively dedicated to vegetables from three-star Michelin chef Alain Passard, you may never eat another vegetable this tasty again.

Musée Rodin
76, Rue de Varenne

Sculptures by Rodin and his contemporaries are on display at his former workshop. A magnificent eighteenth-century mansion with stunning sculpture gardens behind it, it also includes a cute café. Women in Champ de Mars will stop in to roam the quiet gardens and sometimes sit and enjoy a sweet treat. Some of Rodin's most famous works are on-site, including *The Thinker*, *The Kiss*, and *The Gates of Hell*. In *Midnight in Paris*, Owen Wilson and group were led through the gardens by chic Parisian Carla Bruni.

La Pagode
57, Bis Rue de Babylone

A replica of a Chinese pagoda, this classic movie theater, built in 1931, shows special cult classics and art house films. Whether you want to see a film or just need a quiet spot to relax, their lovely tearoom is a quiet retreat.

Coutume Café
47, Rue de Babylone

One of Paris's first of now many high-quality coffee shops, this is where Champ de Mars women stop in for coffee and to read the morning paper. It's a crowded spot for brunch on the weekends, and they're known for their delectable breakfast burrito.

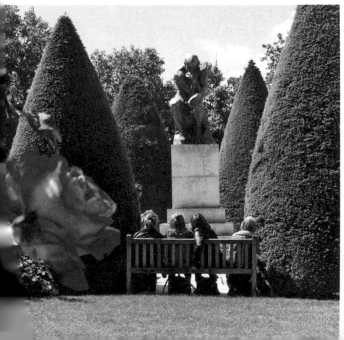
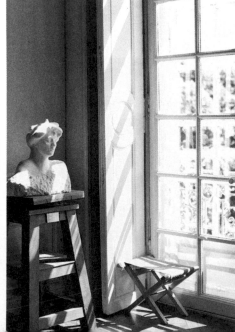
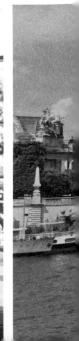

Pont Alexandre III

Although all of the bridges that connect the Right and Left Banks of Paris are unique and beautiful, the Pont Alexandre III, to me, is the most romantic. Connecting Les Invalides with the Grand and Petit Palais, the bridge features art nouveau lamps that light the way of cheerful cherubs, nymphs, and gilded statues.

Hôtel des Invalides and Eglise du Dôme
129, Rue de Grenelle

Walk the grounds of this French military headquarters and the museums dedicated to its history. Enter from Pont Alexandre III to fully appreciate its grandeur and look through the front gardens and you may see a troupe of bunnies hopping around. Inside the church is the tomb of Louis XIV and Napoléon.

Il Vino
13, Boulevard de la Tour-Maubourg

This is the restaurant to bring the wine lovers in your life to. There is no food menu for you to browse over. First, the sommelier will help you select your wine and then the chef will decide what dishes he will cook to best complement your selection. The "blind" tasting menu includes four dishes and four wines.

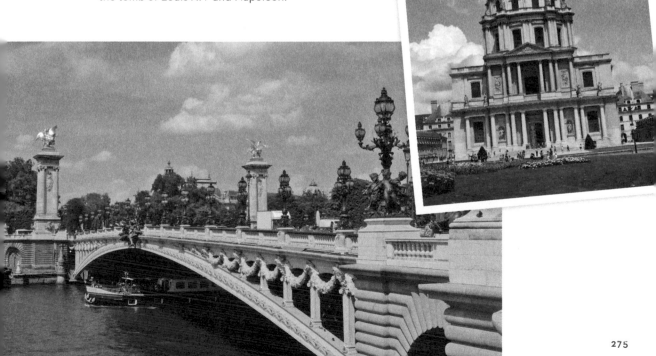

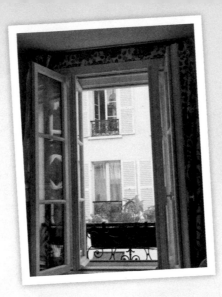

ONE NIGHT IN PARIS

If you only have twenty-four hours to spend in Paris, I can help you make the most of it. Certainly not an ideal timeline, but I know of the most perfect and special location to surround yourself with Parisians and have the best of what Paris has to offer all in one place . . . Hotel Thoumieux.

This boutique hotel is intimate and petite and one of my favorites in which to stay in Paris. Fifteen rooms with the chicest décor, a pâtisserie across the street with delectable pastries, two of Paris's most incredible restaurants creating standout dishes and an unforgettable meal by Chef Jean-François Piège, and last but not least, one of the best views of the Eiffel Tower. Once you've arrived, there's really no need to leave this block on rue Saint-Dominique, except perhaps for a new pair of Christian Louboutin stilettos.

Walk up the steps of this chic hotel and to your right is the dining room of Chef Jean-François Piège's acclaimed two-Michelin-starred Gastronomique. This culinary experience is a once-in-a-lifetime journey where you should savor every last bite.

Have lunch or dinner with girlfriends at Brasserie Thoumieux. It serves the who's who of the neighborhood with incredible signature dishes like Chef Piège's Pizza Soufflé, specially made carbonara, and lemon tart for dessert.

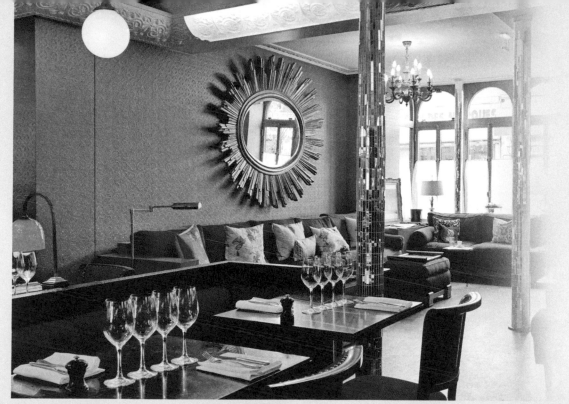

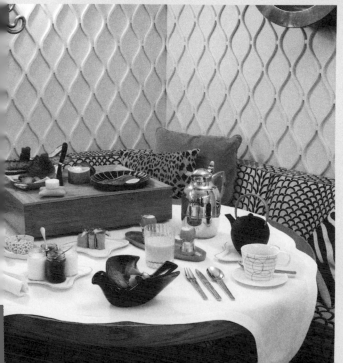

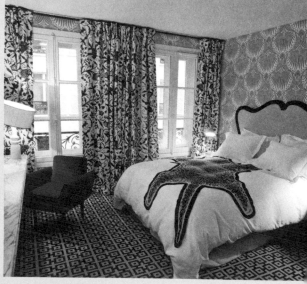

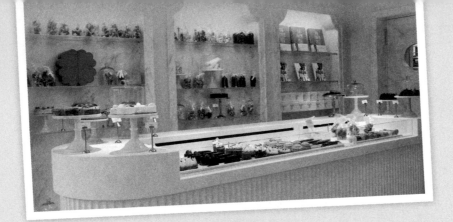

The selection at the Gateaux Thoumieux pâtisserie across the street changes seasonally, with a few signature bites year-round. These are without a doubt some of the best pastries in Paris. You can also take home copies of Chef Piège's cookbooks, homemade jams in adorable jars, homemade marshmallows, and more. There's a new surprise each time I stop in.

Pop outside at night to catch a special city view of the sparkling Eiffel Tower and watch it with Parisians passing by.

Thoumieux, 79, Rue Saint-Dominique

Gateaux Thoumieux, 58, Rue Saint-Dominique

Thoumieux Secret Recipes

Brasserie Thoumieux, with its large banquette tables and modern art deco décor, is one of my favorite restaurants for gossiping with the girls over a tasty lunch or for a big group dinner with friends. Having studied the menu and gotten to know very well their signature dishes, I like to order for the group and surprise my friends with Chef Piège's brasserie classics with his special twist. The group vote is generally that we need only one order of carbonara. That is until it arrives and, after the second or third person has tasted one forkful of the dish with smoked pancetta and egg, it's unanimous that we need to order at least one more. Sometimes not just one, but another two more will do. It's just that delicious and without a doubt the best carbonara that I've ever tasted.

Chef Piège is a very busy man, with his two highly regarded Paris restaurants, a pâtisserie, a hotel, and also a job as host of *Top Chef France*.

He has somehow found the time to compile his signature recipes into a beautiful cookbook with stunning photos. It has been released in English, so you must go to your nearest bookstore to pick up a copy. I feel very honored to be able to share the recipe of my favorite dish at the brasserie. Here, he's left out one special secret ingredient. Try making this at home, and on your next visit to Paris stop in to the brasserie to try his original recipe for yourself.

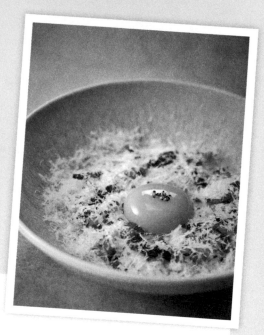

Spaghetti Carbonara

From *Jean-François Piège* by Jean-François Piège

SPAGHETTI DOUGH
- 4 cups wheat flour
- 4 whole eggs
- 5 egg yolks
- 1 tablespoon of water

CARBONARA
- 1/2 pound spaghetti
- 1/4 pound bacon
- 3/4 cups light cream (or half-and-half)
- 3/4 cup grated parmesan cheese
- 1 bunch chopped chives
- Salt, olive oil, freshly ground pepper, to season

To make Spaghetti Dough:

Mix whole eggs and egg yolks in a salad bowl. Add the flour and gradually incorporate the water. When the dough begins to be relatively flexible, flatten it with the palm of the hand to make it homogeneous, then roll it into a ball, Put it in plastic wrap and refrigerate it 2 hours. Roll out spaghetti in a pasta machine.

To make Carbonara

Heat frying pan and cook bacon. Remove from pan, drain, and set aside. Add cream to the pan and slightly reduce. Add the grated Parmesan and set aside.

Boil the water in a pan, salt it, and add a trickle of olive oil. Cook the spaghetti al dente and drain. Toss the pasta in the reduced cream, and add bacon and chopped chives. Place the spaghetti in a deep bowl and make a nest in the center. Gently drop an egg yolk into the nest. Season with salt and freshly ground pepper.

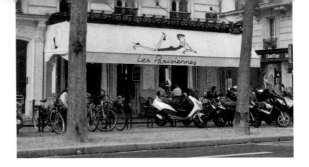

Comptoir de Contonniers
78, Rue Saint-Dominique

Here the Champ de Mars girl finds pieces to put together a look that's "casual chic with a French touch." She'll mix iconic French staples with on-trend silhouettes—a tailored and crisp white button-down, slim-fit jeans, a khaki trench, and a seasonal scarf complete her look for the day. A silk crepe dress over tights is her go-to for night.

Bellota-Bellota
18, Rue Jean-Nicot

The maker of the best Iberian ham in the world. Be prepared, it's melt-in-your-mouth delicious. Pick up slices of ham or order one of their mini tasty sandwiches featuring the ham as the star ingredient. Eat in or take it to go. Champs de Mars ladies stop in on their way to a picnic with family.

L'Ami Jean
27, Rue Maler

Feast on seasonal dishes from the Basque country in southwest France with a heavy focus on wild game. The open kitchen adds a lively environment, fun for group dinners with friends. Reserve the second seating and stay the rest of the night.

Petit Bateau
24, Rue Cler

Petit Bateau has been making the quintessential French striped tees for women, children, and babies for more than one hundred years. So soft and cozy, you need them in every color. The collection has now expanded into ready-to-wear.

Les Parisiennes
17, Avenue de la Motte Picquet

If you're looking for a location to host a girls' brunch, then look no further. Adorable murals inside, a logo of a chic Parisian wearing an LBD and stilettos, and delicious brunch options make this the perfect choice.

Cyrillus
11/13, Avenue Duquesne

Imagine if there were a French version of J. Crew. Imagine no longer—here it is. This casual and versatile collection is French fashion for the entire family.

Les Cocottes
135, Rue Saint-Dominique

A casual eatery by Christian Constant with a key location across from the Eiffel Tower. Your hearty meal of fresh ingredients will arrive in a traditional *cocotte* casserole dish.

Les Fables de la Fontaine
131, Rue Saint-Dominique

Seafood runs deep on this menu and includes everything from sea bass and cod to turbot, langoustines, scallops, and oysters. You can't go wrong by ordering anything on the catch-of-the-day menu.

–Chriselle Lim,
FOUNDER OF THECHRISELLEFACTOR.COM

I never leave Paris without having a picnic under the Eiffel Tower. It's a tradition, and one of my favorite things to do when visiting every year! My favorite memory so far was when my best friend and I got lost in the city. It was past midnight, but we decided not to take a cab and instead find our way back by walking. Although we felt like our feet were going to fall off, we literally saw the entire city that night. We even got to see the Eiffel Tower sparkle at night. The city truly lights up and sparkles at night.

Eiffel Tower

Parisians love to tell you how much they hate *Le Tour Eiffel* and complain about its size and attraction to tourists. However, on occasion, Parisian ladies will admit they do look up when it sparkles and at that point it's a beautiful sight. Don't expect them to ever want to visit the tower with you or go up to the top. I, however, love the sparkles, and no matter how many times I have been lucky enough to watch, I always try to watch again—sometimes going as far as to perch myself on a wall or bench for fifteen or twenty minutes to ensure I catch them and have a great view. You can see the sparkles from many points and areas of Paris, but I won't be sharing my two favorite spots—those are a secret for me and my special someone. You should go to try to find your own.

Now for the important details: It sparkles for five minutes every hour from nightfall until 1 a.m. or 2 a.m., depending on the time of year. If you want to brave the lines to visit and go up the tower, I suggest buying your tickets online in advance and going at sunset for the most beautiful pictures of Paris. Bring a postcard or love letter, which you can leave at the post office located on the second level. It will receive a special stamp only placed on mail sent from that location.

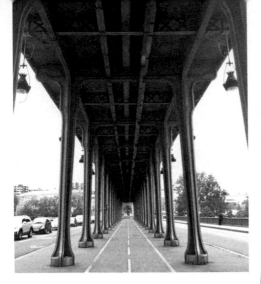

Pont de Bir-Hakeim

This bridge was previously more famous for being the only double-tiered bridge in Paris. It rose to even greater fame when Leonardo DiCaprio it walked across in the film *Inception*. I happen to love it for much more romantic reasons. Although a little more out of the way, it's truly spectacular and magical to walk across. Stop halfway and sit on some of the benches looking out onto the river Seine and the Eiffel Tower.

Maison de la Culture du Japon à Paris
101, Bis Quai Branly

This cultural center showcases Japanese dance performances, both modern and traditional. Make sure to visit on a Wednesday evening for the special tea ceremony.

L'Amaryllis
13, Boulevard Garibaldi

A classic French bistro with classic dishes, such as andouillette and tartare de saumon. Each meal begins with a "panier" of charcuterie and crudité.

CHEESE IF YOU PLEASE

While the 8th arrondissement is known for couture houses and Michelin-starred restaurants, the 7th is touted as having the largest number of award-winning cheese shops in Paris. With half a dozen to choose from, these are a few of my favorites.

FROMAGERIE MARIE-ANNE CANTIN, 12, Rue du Champ de Mars
This unique fromagerie is devoted to cheese in the same way that wine bars are dedicated to their wine. You can shop for cheese, sit for a tasting, and even sign up for courses.

BARTHÉLÉMY, 51, Rue de Grenelle
This shop has been selling more than 250 varieties of cheese since 1904 and even supplies cheese to the homes of the French president and prime minister. Try the specialty soft cheese balls, flavored with cumin and paprika.

LAURENT DUBOIS, 2, Rue de Lourmel
Laurent Dubois has been awarded the highest decoration in *affinage*—the art of cheese ripening and aging—and is known to carry the best Roquefort in Paris. When a Champ de Mars woman is preparing for a dinner party, she orders a platter in advance, which includes handwritten labels to save her time setting up.

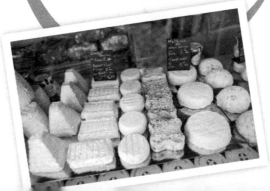

THE FRENCH CHEESE PLATE

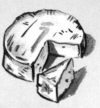

Camembert

One of my most favorite trips to Paris included a day I ventured out of Paris with friends Arielle and Christian and into the vineyards of Burgundy. Just a couple short hours south of Paris, the girls and I spent a glorious day of wine tasting and savored one of the best meals of our lives.

Tomme de Chèvre

That day we encountered our first French cheese course. In most New York restaurants, you create a cheese plate by ordering selections from a menu. No mysteries there. In traditional French restaurants, they bring out an entire cheese plate and leave it with your table. Yes, really. We had no idea what to do, or what the rules and etiquette were. How many cheeses were we allowed to taste? How large a piece? Could we have more than one piece of the same cheese? Could we use the same knife to dip into different cheeses? Too afraid to eat too much and look like greedy Americans, we just savored a small bite of one or two cheeses and left ourselves dreaming of what all the others tasted like. After that meal, I researched the etiquette and asked some Parisian pals for guidance so as to never run into the same dilemma again.

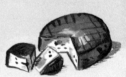

Comte

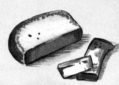

Ossau-Iraty

Here's a helpful cheat sheet:

- Cheeses are arranged clockwise from mildest to strongest and most often begin with a chèvre and end with a blue cheese. Restaurants serve cheese close to its original shape to preserve its taste and prevent it from drying out.

- Choose three to four cheeses to cut from and cut them presentably, so you don't leave the plate in a mess for the next person.

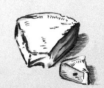

Pont L'Eveque

- Every portion of cheese should contain some of the rind. This will avoid the other tasters being left out, because the taste of the cheese is never always uniform: it gets stronger the closer it is to the rind due to the molding process on the surface.

- There are three types of cheeses in France: goat, sheep, and cow. A few standouts: Tomme de Chèvre (goat), Ossau-Iraty (sheep), and Normandy Camembert (cow).

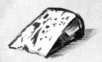

Bleu

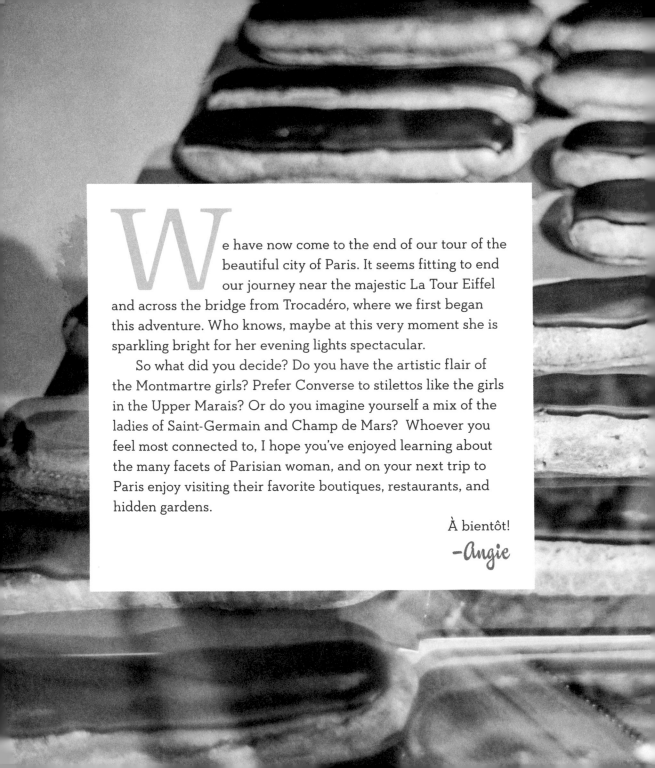

We have now come to the end of our tour of the beautiful city of Paris. It seems fitting to end our journey near the majestic La Tour Eiffel and across the bridge from Trocadéro, where we first began this adventure. Who knows, maybe at this very moment she is sparkling bright for her evening lights spectacular.

So what did you decide? Do you have the artistic flair of the Montmartre girls? Prefer Converse to stilettos like the girls in the Upper Marais? Or do you imagine yourself a mix of the ladies of Saint-Germain and Champ de Mars? Whoever you feel most connected to, I hope you've enjoyed learning about the many facets of Parisian woman, and on your next trip to Paris enjoy visiting their favorite boutiques, restaurants, and hidden gardens.

À bientôt!

—Angie

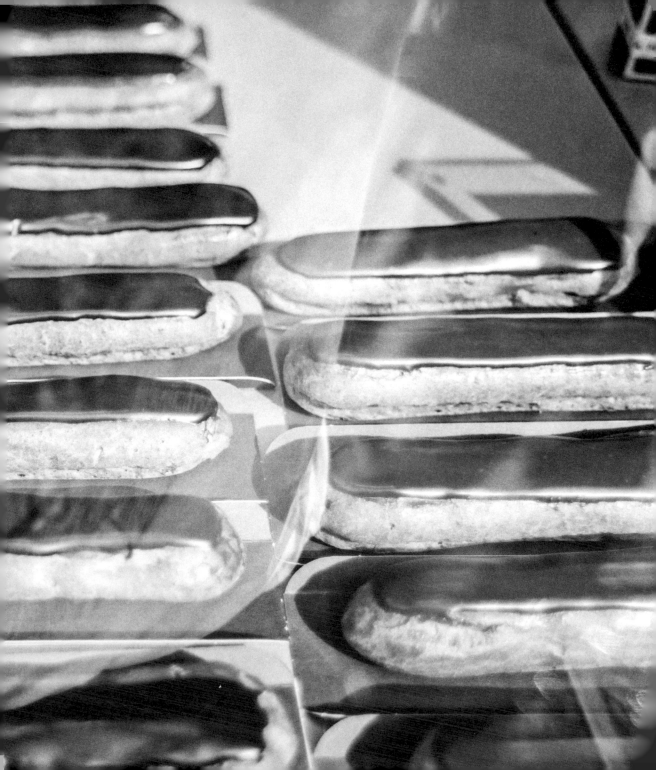

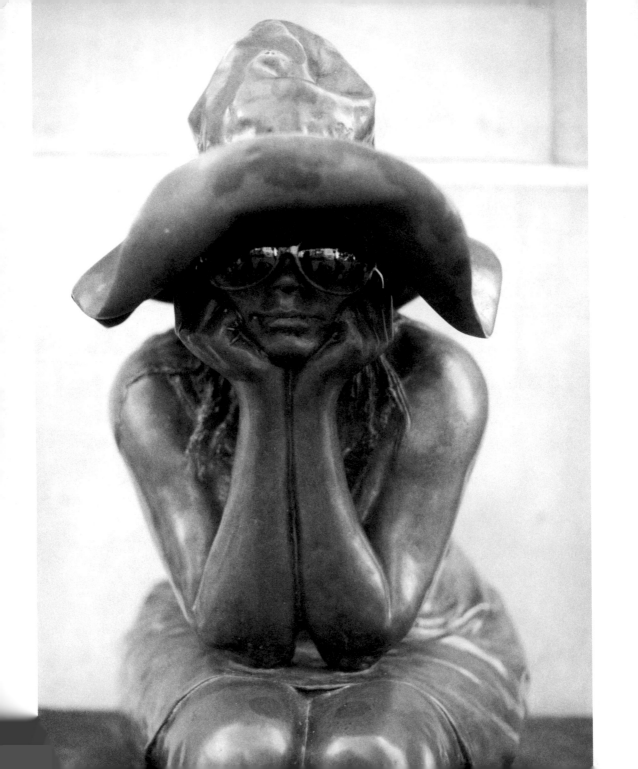

ACKNOWLEDGMENTS

This book is dedicated to my amazing group of girlfriends, most of whom I'm so happy to have shared Parisian adventures (and a few mishaps) with. Thanks for helping me narrow down all of my ideas and putting up with my Paris obsession for so many years. Thank you, Haleigh Walsworth and Keiko Groves for helping me curate the stories with your beautiful photos, and Jason McDonald for literally rolling around on a Parisian street to snap the perfect cover shot. To Iva Zugic, you brought my Parisian girls to life with your lovely illustrations, and your creative vision for the book cover and interiors was beyond inspiring. To the special guy in my life for letting me drag you around Paris over and over when all you wanted to be doing was hanging out in Italy. I love you for that and so much more. To my lit agent, Kim Perel, for your vision and advice in the course of creating the book, and to my editor at Berkley, Denise Silvestro, for making my dream of *Bright Lights Paris* come true. Lastly, to my parents for supporting me through life, school, and an unpaid internship in Paris, which led to my falling head-over-heels in love with the City of Lights.

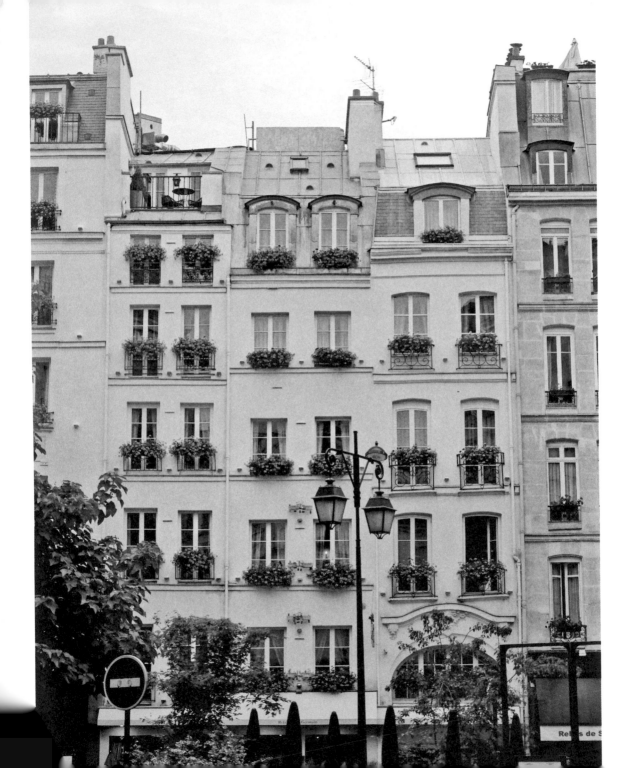

PHOTO AND IMAGE CREDITS

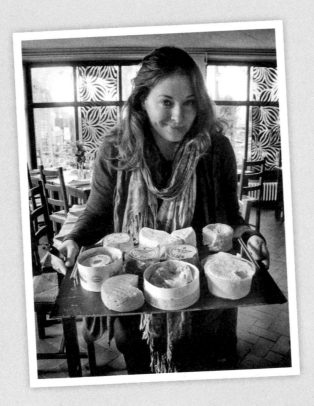

ABOUT THE AUTHOR

A fashion publicist and brand consultant, Angie Niles has worked with some of the biggest names in style—planning red carpet events and fashion shows, international print campaigns, and even dressing some of the worlds chicest stars for the Golden Globes and Oscars. She has lived on both the left and right banks of Paris and now currently resides in Boerum Hill, Brooklyn, or as *Vogue* magazine calls it, "the left bank of New York."

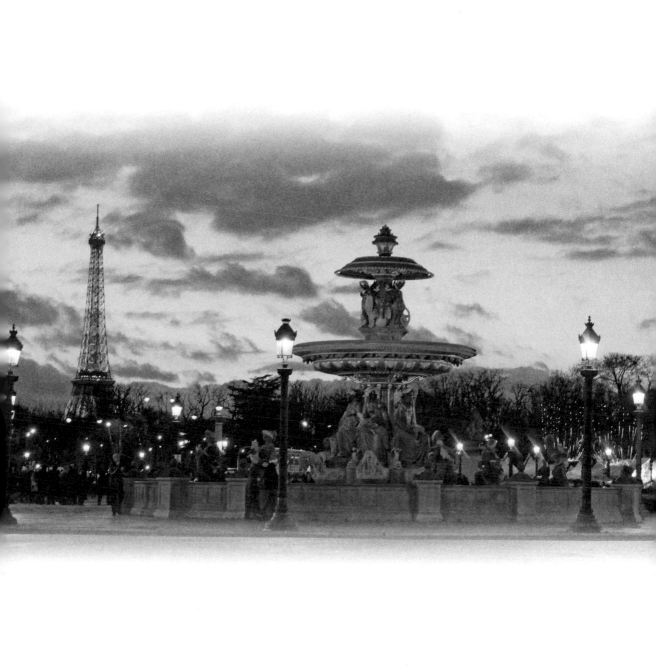

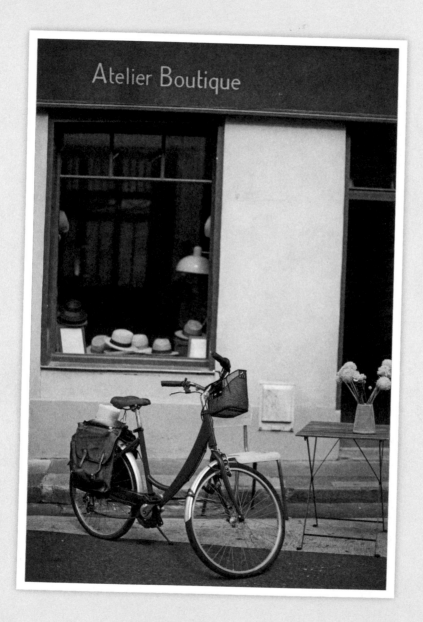